Diabetic Cookbook

Eat healthily to live better

Gena miller

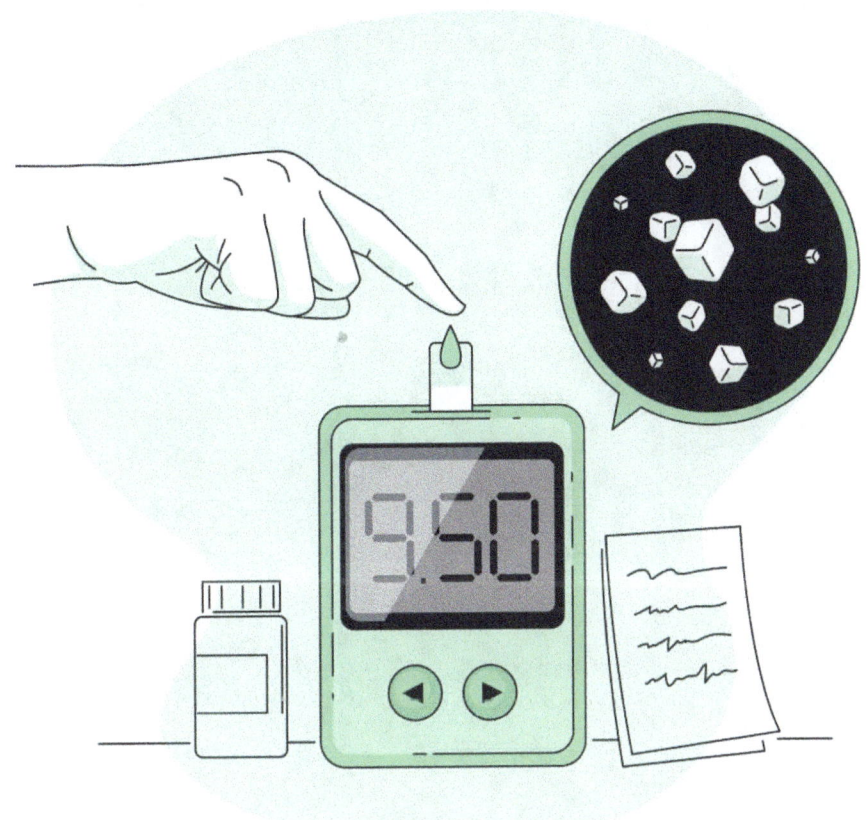

© Copyright 2021 by Gena Miller All rights reserved. The following Book is reproduced below with the goal of providing information that is as accurate and reliable as possible. Regardless, purochasing this Book can be seen as consent to the fact that both the publisher and the author of this book are in no way experts on the topics discussed within and that any recommendations or suggestions that are made herein are for entertainment purposes only. Professionals should be consulted as needed prior to undertaking any of the action endorsed herein. This declaration is deemed fair and valiby both the American Bar Association and the Committee of Publishers Association and is legally binding throughout the United States. Furthermore, the transmission, duplication, or reproduction of any of the following work including specific information will be considered an illegal act irrespective of if it is done electronically or in print. This extends to creating a secondary or tertiary copy of the work or a recorded copy and is only allowed with the express written consent from the Publisher. All additional right reserved. The information in the following pages is broadly considered a truthful and accurate account of facts and as such, any inattention, use, or misuse of the information in question by the reader will render any resulting actions solely under their purview. There are no scenarios in which the publisher or the original author of this work can be in any fashion deemed liable for any hardship or damages that may befall them after undertaking information described herein.! & Additionally, the information in the following pages is intended only for informational purposes and should thus be thought of as universal. As befitting its nature, it is presented without assurance regarding its prolonged validity or interim quality. Trademarks that are mentioned are done without written consent and can in no way be considered an endorsement from the trademark holder.

Table of content

Breakfast 18
Avocado Goat Cheese Toast 20
Brussels Sprout Hash with Eggs 20
Zucchini Bread 21
Broccoli and Mushroom Frittata 22
Ratatouille Egg Bake 23
Banana Crêpe Cakes 24
Mushroom & Asparagus Frittata 25
Fish Simmered In Tomato-Pepper Sauce 26
Salad With Ranch 27
Mustard Chicken 27
Stylish Chicken-Bacon Wrap 28
Whole Egg Baked Sweet Potatoes 29
Quinoa Burrito 31
Chicken and Egg Salad 31
Tex-Mex Migas 32
Yogurt Sundae 33
Breakfast Egg Bites 34
Savory Corn Grits 35
Blueberry Coconut Breakfast Cookies 35
Toads in Holes 36
Walnut and Oat Granola 37
Apple and Bran Muffins 38
Greek Yogurt and Oat Pancakes 39

Asparagus Frittata 40
Whole-Grain Dutch Baby Pancake 41
Lovely Porridge 42
Greek Chicken Breast 42
Breakfast Salad 43
Cheese Yogurt 44
Breakfast Cake 44
Lunch 47
Brunswick Stew 49
Chicken Chili 50
Chicken and Pepperoni 51
Comforting Summer Squash Soup with Crispy Chickpeas 52
Arugula and Avocado Salad 53
Bean and Scallion Salad 53
Chicken Vera Cruz 55
Fire-Roasted Tomatoes Over Chicken 56
Vegetable Minestrone Soup 57
Three-Pepper Pizza 58
Parmesan Baked Cod 58
Cilantro Lime Shrimp 59
Turkey Coriander Dish 60
Lentil And Eggplant Stew 60
Eggplant Curry 61
Blueberry and Chicken Salad 61
Buffalo Chicken Salads 63
Chicken and Cornmeal Dumplings 64
Moroccan Eggplant Stew 65

Crispy Dill Salmon 67
Green Salad with Berries and Sweet Potatoes 68
Blueberry and Chicken Salad 69
Buffalo Chicken Salads 69
Orange Chicken Thighs 70
Artichoke Ratatouille Chicken 71
Vegan Chili with White Bean 72
Roasted Chickpea in Curry Bowl 73
Pepper Steak Squash 74
Flank Steak Beef 75
French Onion Soup 76
Dinner 78
Herbed Chicken Meal 80
Italian Pork Chops 81
Baked Broccoli Chicken 82
Chicken breast on vegetable noodles 83
Grilled Steak Pinwheels 84
Taco-stuffed Peppers 84
Quinoa Cakes with Fresh Tomato–cilantro Sauce 85
Shrimp Salad 87
Summer Spinach Salad with Grilled Chicken and Creamy 87
Greek Style Quesadillas 88
Creamy Penne 89
Colourful Tuna Salad with Bocconcini 90
Baked Eggplant Turkey 91
Turkey Sausages 92
Baked Garlic Lemon Salmon 92

Hearty Pumpkin Chicken Soup 94
Colorful sweet potato salad 95
Barbecue Pork Loin 96
Ginger Halibut Bites 97
Sirloin Steak With Tomato & Pepper 98
Italian Chicken 99
Parmesan-Topped Acorn Squash 100
Fish & Chip Traybake 101
Pork in Chinese 102
Coconut Chicken Curry 102
Chicken and Veggie Soup 103
Seafood and Andouille Medley 104
Chicken and Veggie Soup 105
Ground Lamb with Peas 105
Asian-Style Pan-Fried Chicken 106
Dessert 109
Strawberry Lemon Muffins 111
English Muffins 112
Chocolate Cookies 112
Coconut Keto Bombs 113
Pecan Coffee Cake 114
Jalapeno and Cheddar Muffins 115
Honey Raisin Cookies 116
Sweet Potato Bread 117
Raspberry and Cashew Balls 118
Conclusion 120

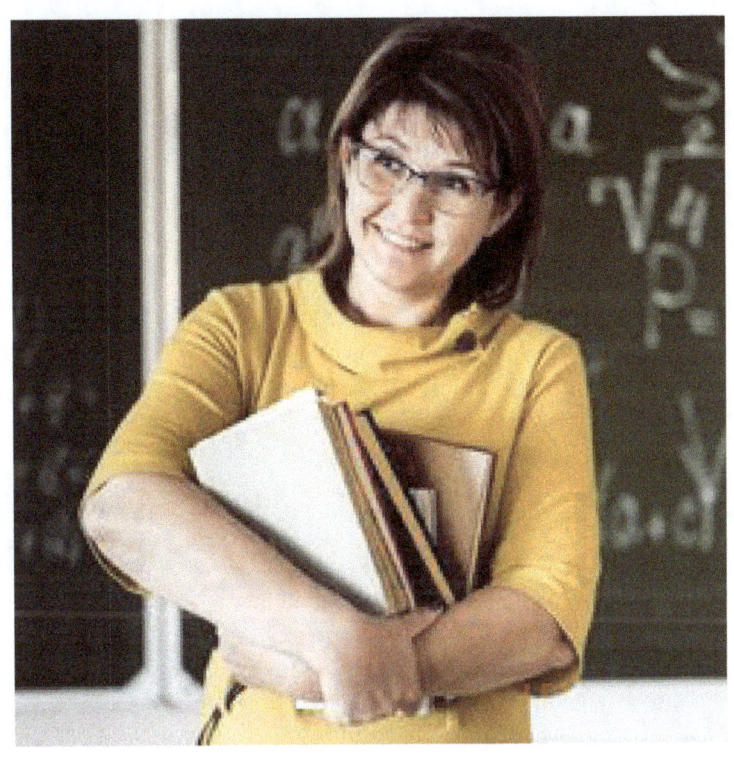

Gena Miller was born in Portland Oregon in 1970 to a wealthy family, Gena has the opportunity to continue her studies away from home, thanks to the economic aid of her father, and for this reason, she decided to attend the renowned university "Columbia University in New York". She had no difficulty in graduating in 1998 with top marks, winning a scholarship in "nutritional sciences" which allowed her to find a job at the university as a lecturer. Gena took her profession very much to heart and saw in teaching the possibility of giving her students the necessary tools to establish a healthy and wholesome lifestyle, drawing up for them real nutritional plans with tasty and healthy recipes. It was her students who encouraged her to start writing "health and wellness" books. The first books were a success and were a stimulus for many people so Gena soon became a successful writer, her experience and love for others led her to understand the real needs of people with food problems and the difficulties they had in approaching food, Gena managed more and more to give the right amount of nutritional value and good taste to her dishes creating delicious and easy recipes appreciated by all.

Introduction

Diabetes is a disease that affects many people, and there are those of us who deal with it on a daily basis. Having diabetes can be difficult for a number of reasons. For one, you have to constantly watch what you eat, and this can get very tedious. In fact, you also have to be very careful about the amount of carbohydrates you eat. If you're not careful, this can have a negative effect on your health and can even alter your mood, which is never good. To control diabetes and its many side effects, you need to make sure that you have a healthy diet plan that is easy to follow. In many cases, dehydration occurs as a result of vomiting and diarrhea. Diabetics may only notice dehydration when their urine turns a darker color. One thing that affects the blood sugar level of diabetic patients is their diet. People who have diabetes should stay away from foods with a high glycemic index, such as those made from corn, wheat and rice, because these foods can raise blood sugar levels quickly. Low glycemic index foods include all fruits, which means you can eat them without your blood sugar levels rising quickly. Foods like Greek yogurt tend to have a lower glycemic index, so if you are diabetic and need to avoid high glycemic index foods, Greek yogurt can be your best friend. There are many different ways that people can treat diabetes, however the one thing that could be done to help most with diabetes would be to lower it through diet and exercise. Both of these things will work in conjunction with each other to help lower blood sugar levels. In order to lower your blood sugar as much as possible, a look at your diet is important because what you eat greatly affects how your blood sugar levels work. How you maintain your weight also plays an important role in how your diabetes works and may even have a positive effect on it. Whatever the connotation of diet and diabetes, it's important to understand that there aren't many things you can do to treat the disease. What you can do is try to manage it as best you can with a healthy diet, and then get plenty of exercise. Not only should you deal with your diabetes through treatment, but you should also make sure that it doesn't cause other health problems like high cholesterol levels or the risk of heart disease. There are many different ways to treat diabetes, however the one thing that could be done to help most diabetics would be to lower it through diet and exercise. Both of these things will work in conjunction with each other to help lower the blood sugar level. In order to lower your blood sugar as much as possible, a look at your diet is important because what you eat greatly affects how your blood sugar levels work. How you maintain your weight also plays an important role in how your diabetes works and may even have a positive effect on it. Since diabetes is primarily caused by lifestyle factors, it is essential to manage the disease through proper diet and exercise. Diet and exercise together can ensure you are at a healthy weight that will help prevent the high blood glucose levels that come with diabetes. Your doctor will be able to tell you more about the appropriate diet for you. If you are overweight, you should lose weight. If you are not overweight but have excess fat, you should avoid gaining weight or maintain your current weight. This can be done through portion control and choosing healthy foods. For the main part, a healthy, balanced diet can help with diabetes. A healthy mix of carbohydrates, proteins and fats is usually recommended for people with diabetes. It is important not to avoid sugar completely when trying to treat diabetes. While sugar can be part of a diet that is healthy for people with diabetes, it should be used in moderation. Exercising regularly while controlling what you eat will help you maintain a healthy weight and will also help your blood sugar levels stay under control since the food you eat will stay in a normal range instead of going high or low.

Breakfast

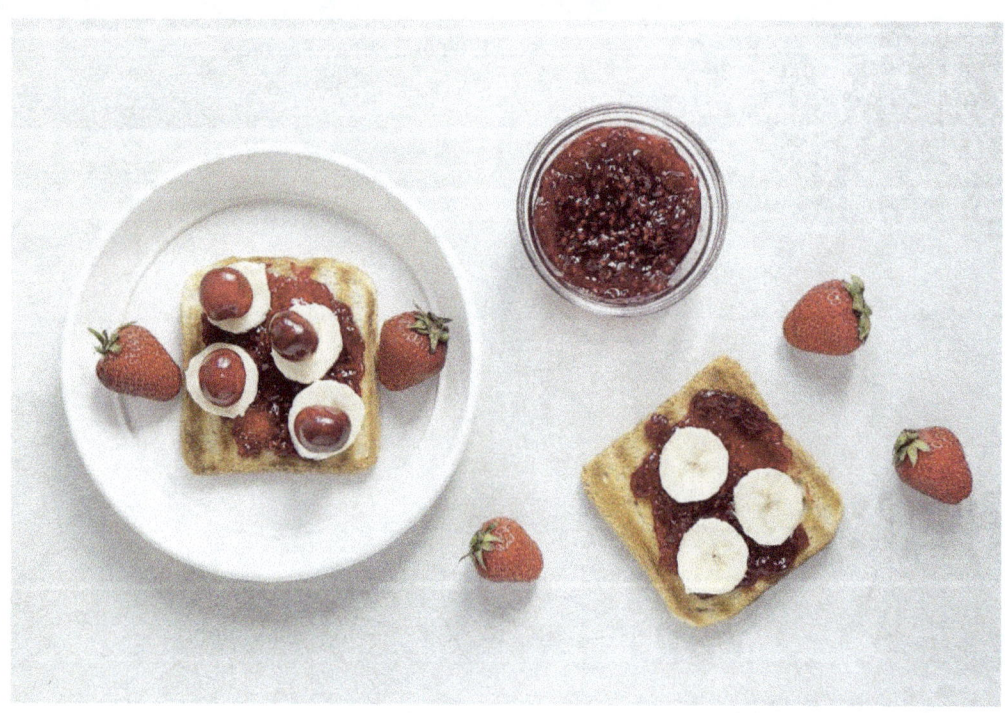

Avocado Goat Cheese Toast

Nutrition facts: calories: 137 | fat: 6g | protein: 5g | carbs: 18g | sugars: 0g | fiber: 5g | sodium: 195mg

Prep time: 5 minutes

Cook time: 10 minutes

Serves 2

Ingredients:

- 2 slices whole-wheat thin-sliced bread
- ½ avocado
- 2 tablespoons crumbled goat cheese
- Salt, to taste

Instruction:

1. In a toaster or broiler, toast the bread until browned.
2. Remove the flesh from the avocado.
3. In a medium bowl, use a fork to mash the avocado flesh.
4. Spread it onto the toast.
5. Sprinkle with the goat cheese and season lightly with salt.
6. Add any toppings and serve.

Brussels Sprout Hash with Eggs

Prep time: 15 minutes

Cook time: 15 minutes

Serves 4

Ingredients:

- 3 teaspoons extra-virgin olive oil,
- divided 1 pound (454 g) Brussels sprouts,
- sliced 2 garlic cloves,
- thinly sliced ¼ teaspoon salt Juice of 1 lemon
- 4 eggs In a large skillet,
- heat 1½ teaspoons of oil over medium heat.

Instructions:

1. Add the Brussels sprouts and toss.
2. Cook, stirring regularly, for 6 to 8 minutes until browned and softened.
3. Add the garlic and continue to cook until fragrant, about 1 minute.
4. Season with the salt and lemon juice.
5. Transfer to a serving dish.
6. In the same pan, heat the remaining 1½ teaspoons of oil over medium-high heat.
7. Crack the eggs into the pan.
8. Fry for 2 to 4 minutes, flip, and continue cooking to desired doneness.
9. Serve over the bed of hash.

Nutrition facts: Per Serving calories: 158 | fat: 9g | protein: 10g | carbs: 12g | sugars: 4g | fiber: 4g | sodium: 234mg

Zucchini Bread

Prep time: 15 minute

Cook time: 45 minutes

Serves 24

Ingredients:

- 1½ cups gluten-free all-purpose flour
- 1 cup almond meal
- ½ cup chickpea flour
- 1 teaspoon salt
- 1 teaspoon baking powder
- 1 teaspoon baking soda
- ½ teaspoon ground nutmeg
- ½ teaspoon ground cinnamon
- 3 medium brown eggs
- ¼ cup sunflower seed oil
- 2 ripe bananas,

Instructions:

1. mashed 2 zucchini, grated, with water squeezed out 2 teaspoons almond extract

2. Preheat the oven to 350°F (180°C).
3. Line a 9 × 13-inch pan with parchment paper.
4. In a large bowl, use a fork or whisk to combine the gluten-free flour, almond meal, chickpea flour, salt, baking powder, baking soda, nutmeg, and cinnamon.
5. In a separate large bowl, beat the eggs, oil, bananas, zucchini, and almond extract together well.
6. Fold the dry ingredients into the wet ingredients, stir until well combined, and pour into the prepared pan.
7. Transfer the pan to the oven, and bake for 40 to 45 minutes, or until a butter knife inserted into the center comes out clean.
8. Remove from the oven, and let the bread rest for 15 minutes before serving.

Nutrition facts: Per Serving calories: 203 | fat: 11g | protein: 6g | carbs: 21g | sugars: 4g | fiber: 4g | sodium: 323mg

Broccoli and Mushroom Frittata

Prep time: 5 minutes

Cook time: 10 minutes

Serves 4

Ingredients:

- 2 tablespoons extra-virgin olive oil
- ½ onion, finely chopped
- 1 cup broccoli florets
- 1 cup sliced shiitake mushrooms
- 1 garlic clove,
- minced 8 large eggs, beaten
- ½ teaspoon sea salt
- ½ cup grated Parmesan cheese

Instructions:

1. Preheat the oven broiler on high.
2. In a medium ovenproof skillet over medium-high heat, heat the olive oil until it shimmers.

3. Add the onion, broccoli, and mushrooms, and cook, stirring occasionally, until the vegetables start to brown, about 5 minutes.
4. Add the garlic and cook, stirring constantly, for 30 seconds.
5. Arrange the vegetables in an even layer on the bottom of the pan.
6. While the vegetables cook, in a small bowl, whisk together the eggs and salt.
7. Carefully pour the eggs over the vegetables.
8. Cook without stirring, allowing the eggs to set around the vegetables.
9. As the eggs begin to set around the edges, use a spatula to pull the edges away from the sides of the pan.
10. Tilt the pan and allow the uncooked eggs to run into the spaces.
11. Cook 1 to 2 minutes more, until it sets around the edges.
12. The eggs will still be runny on top.
13. Sprinkle with the Parmesan and place the pan in the broiler.
14. Broil until brown and puffy, about 3 minutes.
15. Cut into wedges to serve.

Nutrition facts: Per Serving calories: 280 | fat: 21g | protein: 19g | carbs: 7g | sugars: 1g | fiber: 2g | sodium: 654mg

Ratatouille Egg Bake

Prep time: 20 minutes

Cook time: 50 minutes

Serves: 4

Ingredients:

- 2 teaspoons extra-virgin olive oil
- ½ sweet onion, finely chopped
- 2 teaspoons minced garlic
- ½ small eggplant, peeled and diced
- 1 green zucchini, diced
- 1 yellow zucchini, diced
- 1 red bell pepper, seeded and diced
- 3 tomatoes, seeded and chopped
- 1 tablespoon chopped fresh oregano

- 1 tablespoon chopped fresh basil
- Pinch red pepper flakes
- Sea salt and freshly ground black pepper, to taste
- 4 large eggs

Instructions:

1. Preheat the oven to 350°F (180°C).
2. Place a large ovenproof skillet over medium heat and add the olive oil.
3. Sauté the onion and garlic until softened and translucent, about 3 minutes.
4. Stir in the eggplant and sauté for about 10 minutes, stirring occasionally.
5. Stir in the zucchini and pepper and sauté for 5 minutes.
6. Reduce the heat to low and cover
7. Cook until the vegetables are soft, about 15 minutes.
8. Stir in the tomatoes, oregano, basil, and red pepper flakes, and cook 10 minutes more.
9. Season the ratatouille with salt and pepper.
10. Use a spoon to create four wells in the mixture.
11. Crack an egg into each well.
12. Place the skillet in the oven and bake until the eggs are firm, about 5 minutes.
13. Remove from the oven.
14. Serve the eggs with a generous scoop of vegetables.

Nutrition facts: per Serving: calories: 148 fat: 7.9g protein: 9.1g carbs: 13.1g fiber: 4.1g sugar: 7.1g sodium: 99mg

Banana Crêpe Cakes

Prep time: 5 minutes

Cook time: 20 minutes

Serves: 4

Ingredients:

- Avocado oil cooking spray
- 4 ounces (113 g) reduced-fat plain cream cheese, softened
- 2 medium bananas
- 4 large eggs
- ½ teaspoon vanilla extract
- 1/8 teaspoon salt

Instructions:

1. Heat a large skillet over low heat.
2. Coat the cooking surface with cooking spray, and allow the pan to heat for another 2 to 3 minutes.
3. Meanwhile, in a medium bowl, mash the cream cheese and bananas together with a fork until combined.
4. The bananas can be a little chunky.
5. Add the eggs, vanilla, and salt, and mix well.
6. For each cake, drop 2 tablespoons of the batter onto the warmed skillet and use the bottom of a large spoon or ladle to spread it thin.
7. Let it cook for 7 to 9 minutes
8. Flip the cake over and cook briefly, about 1 minute.

Nutrition facts: per Serving: calories: 176 fat: 9.1g protein: 9.1g carbs: 15.1g fiber: 2.1g sugar: 8.1g sodium: 214mg

Mushroom & Asparagus Frittata

Prep time: 10 minutes

Cook time: 13 minutes

Serves: 4

Ingredients:

- 1 cup mushrooms, fresh chopped
- 1 cup asparagus, fresh-cut
- ½ cup broccoli florets, chopped
- ¼ cup nonfat milk
- 3 egg whites
- 3 eggs
- ½ teaspoon of sea salt
- 1/8 teaspoon crushed red pepper
- 1 clove garlic, minced
- ½ red bell pepper, chopped
- 2 scallions, thinly sliced

Instructions:

1. Coat a nonstick large skillet with some cooking spray, then heat over the medium-high heat.

2. Add the mushrooms, asparagus, broccoli, scallions, garlic, bell pepper, crushed red pepper and salt.
3. Cook for approximately 3 minutes, or until your vegetables are tender.
4. In a mixing bowl, whisk your whole egg whites, eggs, and milk.
5. Next, reduce the skillet to medium-low and then add in the egg mixture.
6. As the egg mixture begins to set, push cooked edges slightly towards the center; this will allow the liquid to run to the edges of skillet.
7. Reduce the heat to low and cover skillet; continue to cook for an additional 10 minutes or until the eggs are set.
8. Slide the frittata onto a serving platter.
9. Slice into four wedges.
10. Serve and enjoy!

Nutritional facts: (per ½ recipe): Calories: 93 Fat: 4g Protein: 10g Carbs: 5g

Fish Simmered In Tomato-Pepper Sauce

Prep time: 5 min

Cook time: 10 min

Serves: 3

Ingredients:

- 2 (4-oz) cod fillets (or another firm, white fish)
- 1 big tomato
- 1/3 cup red peppers (roasted)
- 3 tbsp almonds
- 2 cloves garlic
- 2 tbsp fresh basil leaves
- 1 or 2 tbsp extra virgin olive oil
- 1/4 tsp salt
- 1/8 tsp pepper

Instructions:

1. Toast sliced almonds in a pan until fragrant.
2. Grind almonds, basil, minced garlic, 1-2 tsp oil in a food processor until finely ground.
3. Add coarsely-chopped tomato and red peppers; grind until smooth.

4. Season fish with salt and pepper.
5. Cook in hot oil in a large pan over medium-high heat until fish is browned.
6. Pour sauce around fish.

Nutrition facts: (100 g) Calories 90 Protein 8 g Fat 5 g Carbs 7 g

1. Combine chopped lettuce, chopped cucumber, and halved tomatoes in a bowl.
2. Drizzle with dressing, and sprinkle with pepper.
3. Toss.

Nutrition facts: (100 g) Calories 80 Protein 12 g Fat 2 g Carbs 0,1 g

Salad With Ranch

Prep time: 10 min

Cook time: 0 min

Serving: 1

Ingredients:

1. 1/2 (10-oz) pkg iceberg lettuce
2. 1/2 cup cucumber
3. 1/4 cup grape tomatoes
4. 2 tbsp refrigerated yogurt (sugar-free)
5. 1/4 tsp pepper

Instructions:

Mustard Chicken

Prep Time: 10 minutes

Cook Time: 40 minutes

Serves: 4

Ingredients:

- 4 chicken breasts
- 1/2 cup chicken broth
- 3-4 tablespoons mustard
- 3 tablespoons olive oil
- 1 teaspoon paprika
- 1 teaspoon chili powder
- 1 teaspoon garlic powder

Instructions:

1. Take a small bowl and mix mustard, olive oil, paprika, chicken broth, garlic powder, chicken broth, and chili
2. Add chicken breast and marinate for 30 minutes
3. Take a lined baking sheet and arrange the chicken
4. Bake for 35 minutes at 375 degrees Fahrenheit
5. Serve and enjoy!

Nutrition facts: Calories: 531; Fat: 23g; Carbohydrates: 10g; Protein: 64g

Stylish Chicken-Bacon Wrap

Prep Time: 5 minutes

Cook Time: 50 minutes

Serves: 3

Ingredients:

- 8 ounces lean chicken breast
- 6 bacon slices
- 3 ounces shredded cheese
- 4 slices ham

Instructions:

1. Cut chicken breast into bite-sized portions
2. Transfer shredded cheese onto ham slices
3. Roll up chicken breast and ham slices in bacon slices
4. Take a skillet and place it over medium heat
5. Add olive oil and brown bacon for a while
6. Remove rolls and transfer to your oven
7. Bake for 45 minutes at 325 degrees F

8. Serve and enjoy!

Nutrition facts: Calories: 275; Fat: 11g; Carbohydrates: 0.5g; Protein: 40g

Whole Egg Baked Sweet Potatoes

Prep Time: 30 minutes

Cook Time: 60 minutes

Serves: 4

Ingredients:

For the Potatoes:

- 4 medium sweet potatoes
- 2 heads garlic
- 2 tsp. extra virgin olive oil
- ½ tbsp. taco Seasoning
- ¼ cup fresh cilantro, plus additional for garnish
- Salt and pepper
- 4 eggs

For the Sauce:

- ½ cup avocado, about 1 medium avocado
- 1 tbsp. fresh lime juice
- 1 tsp. lime zest
- Salt and pepper
- 2 tbsp. water

Instructions:

1. Preheat the oven to 395°F, cover with a baking sheet and tinfoil then place the potatoes on it.
2. Rip off the garlic tips, keep the head intact, and softly rub in the olive oil on top of the uncovered cloves.
3. Create 2 layers of tinfoil in a small packet and wrapping the garlic in it, then put it in the pan.
4. Bake the garlic for about 40 minutes, until it is tender.
5. Remove from the pan and proceed to cook the potatoes for additional 25–35 minutes, until fork-tender and soft.
6. When the potatoes are tender, set them aside for about 10 minutes until they're cool enough to treat.
7. In addition, decrease the temperature of the oven to 375°F.

8. Break the potatoes down the middle and softly peel the skin back, leaving the skin intact on the sides.
9. In a wide cup, carefully scoop out the skin, leaving a little amount on the sides of the potato to help maintain its form.
10. Mash the flesh of the sweet potato and then cut half of it from the bowl (you will not use this flesh, so use it at a later date in another meal!) Add in the taco seasoning, cilantro and season with salt and pepper to taste into the mashed flesh.
11. Finally, from the roasted heads, squeeze in all the fluffy garlic.
12. Blend well.
13. Divide the flesh between the 4 sweet potatoes, spreading it softly to fill the meat, leaving a large hole in the middle of each potato.
14. Back on the baking sheet, put the sweet potatoes and crack an egg into each hole and spray it with pepper and salt.
15. Bake to your taste until the egg is well fried.
16. For a good runny yolk, it normally takes about 10–15 minutes and blend until smooth.
17. Then, with the food processor running, pour in the water and combine until well mixed.
18. Sprinkle with salt and pepper to taste.
19. Break the avocado sauce between them until the potatoes are cooked, spreading it out on top.
20. Garnish with sliced tomatoes and cilantro in addition.
21. And enjoy!

Nutrition facts: Calories: 399 Fat: 32g Protein: 18g

Quinoa Burrito

Prep Time: 15 minutes

Cook Time: 10 minutes

Serves: 1

Ingredients:

- 1 cup quinoa
- 2 cups black beans
- 4 finely chopped onions, green
- 4 finely chopped garlic
- 2 freshly cut limes
- 1 big tbsp. cumin
- 2 beautifully diced avocado
- 1 small cup beautifully diced cilantro

Instructions:

1. Boil quinoa.
2. During this process, put the beans in low heat.
3. Add other ingredients to the bean pot and let it mix well for about 15 minutes.
4. Serve quinoa and add the prepared beans.

Nutrition facts: Calories: 117 Protein: 27g Fiber: 10g

Chicken and Egg Salad

Prep Time: 5 minutes

Cook Time: 25 minutes

Serves: 2

Ingredients:

- 2 cooked chicken breasts
- 3 hard-boiled eggs
- 2 tbsp. fat-free mayo
- 1 tbsp. curry powder
- Chives or basil (optional)
- Salt (optional)

Instructions:

1. Bake the chicken for maybe 15 minutes in the oven around 360°F (confirm with just a knife that now the meat is cooked all the through).
2. For 8 minutes, cook the eggs.

3. Cut the eggs and chicken into a small-sized piece.
4. Combine the cream cheese with curry powder
5. In a large bowl, combine everything and mix.
6. Allow a minimum of 10 minutes to chill in the refrigerator (it gets even better if you leave it overnight in the refrigerator).
7. Serve with chives on toast or muffins and a bit of salt on top.

Nutrition facts: Calories: 139 Fat 9g Carbohydrate: 23g

Tex-Mex Migas

Prep Time: 9 minutes

Cook Time: 15 minutes

Serves: 4

Ingredients:

- 3 large eggs
- 3 egg whites
- 1 tbsp. canola oil
- 4 corn tortillas, cut into ½-inch-wide strips
- ½ cup chopped onion
- 2 large seeded jalapeño peppers
- 2-third cup lower-sodium salsa
- ½ cup Monterey Jack cheese, shredded
- ½ cup sliced green onions
- Hot sauce (optional)
- Lower-sodium red salsa (optional)
- Lower-sodium green salsa (optional)

Instruction:

1. Place the eggs and egg whites in a bowl; stir until mixed with a whisk.

2. Over medium-high prepare, heat a medium nonstick skillet.
3. In a bath, apply oil; swirl to coat.
4. Apply tortilla strips to the skillet and cook, stirring constantly, for 3 minutes or until brown.
5. In a sauce, add the onion and jalapeño peppers; sauté for 2 minutes or until tender.
6. Stir in 2/3 of a cup salsa, and simmer for 1 minute, stirring continuously.
7. Add the mixture of eggs; simmer for 2 minutes or until the eggs are tender, stirring periodically.
8. Sprinkle the cheese with the egg mixture.
9. Cook for thirty seconds or until the cheese is molten.
10. Cover with the green onions, then serve right away.
11. If preferred, serve with hot sauce, red salsa, or green salsa.

Nutrition facts: Calories: 193 Fat: 10.4g Protein: 10.2g

Yogurt Sundae

Prep time: 5 minutes

Cook time: 0 minutes

Serves 1

Ingredients:

- ¾ cup plain nonfat Greek yogurt
- ¼ cup mixed berries (blueberries, strawberries, blackberries)
- 2 tablespoons cashew, walnut, or almond pieces
- 1 tablespoon ground flaxseed
- 2 fresh mint leaves,

Instruction:

1. shredded Spoon the yogurt into a small bowl.
2. Top with the berries, nuts, and flaxseed.
3. Garnish with the mint and serve.

Nutrition fats : calories: 238 | fat: 11g | protein: 21g | carbs: 16g | sugars: 9g | fiber: 4g | sodium: 64mg

Breakfast Egg Bites

Prep time: 10 minutes

Cook time: 25 minutes

Serves 8

Ingredients:

- Nonstick cooking spray 6 eggs, beaten
- ¼ cup unsweetened plain almond milk
- 1 red bell pepper, diced
- 1 cup chopped spinach
- ¼ cup crumbled goat cheese
- ½ cup sliced brown mushrooms
- ¼ cup sliced sun-dried tomatoes Salt and freshly ground black pepper, to taste

Instructions:

1. Preheat the oven to 350°F (180°C).
2. Spray 8 muffin cups of a 12-cup muffin tin with nonstick cooking spray.
3. Set aside.
4. In a large mixing bowl, combine the eggs, almond milk, bell pepper, spinach, goat cheese, mushrooms, and tomatoes.
5. Season with salt and pepper.
6. Fill the prepared muffin cups three-fourths full with the egg mixture.
7. Bake for 20 to 25 minutes until the eggs are set.
8. Let cool slightly and remove the egg bites from the muffin tin.
9. Serve warm, or store in an airtight container in the refrigerator for up to 5 days or in the freezer for up to 1 month.

Nutrition facts: Per Serving calories: 68 | fat: 4g | protein: 6g | carbs: 3g | sugars: 2g | fiber: 1g | sodium: 126mg

Savory Corn Grits

Prep time: 5 minutes

Cook time: 7 minutes

Serves 4

Ingredients:

- 2 cups water
- 1 cup fat-free milk
- 1 cup stone-ground corn grits

Instructions:

1. In a heavy-bottomed pot, bring the water and milk to a simmer over medium heat.
2. Gradually add the grits, stirring continuously.
3. Reduce the heat to low, cover, and cook, stirring often, for 5 to 7 minutes, or until the grits are soft and tender.
4. Serve and enjoy.

Nutrition facts: Per Serving calories: 166 | fat: 1g | protein: 6g | carbs: 34g | sugars: 3g | fiber: 1g | sodium: 32mg

Blueberry Coconut Breakfast Cookies

Prep time: 10 minutes

Cook time: 15 minutes

Serves 4

Ingredients:

- 4 tablespoons unsalted butter, at room temperature
- 2 medium bananas
- 4 large eggs
- ½ cup unsweetened applesauce
- 1 teaspoon vanilla extract
- ⅔ cup coconut flour ¼ teaspoon salt
- 1 cup fresh or frozen blueberries

Instructions:

1. Preheat the oven to 375°F (190°C).
2. In a medium bowl, mash the butter and bananas together with a fork until combined.
3. The bananas can be a little chunky.

4. Add the eggs, applesauce, and vanilla to the bananas and mix well.
5. Stir in the coconut flour and salt.
6. Gently fold in the blueberries.
7. Drop about 2 tablespoons of dough on a baking sheet for each cookie and flatten it a bit with the back of a spoon.
8. Bake for about 13 minutes, or until firm to the touch.

Nutrition facts: Per Serving calories: 305 | fat: 18g | protein: 8g | carbs: 28g | sugars: 15g | fiber: 7g | sodium: 222mg

Toads in Holes

Prep time: 5 minutes

Cook time: 5 minutes

Serves 2

Ingredients:

- 2 tablespoons butter
- 2 slices whole-wheat bread
- 2 large eggs

Instructions:

1. Sea salt and freshly ground black pepper, to taste In a medium nonstick skillet over medium heat, heat the butter until it bubbles.
2. As the butter heats, cut a 3-inch hole in the middle of each piece of bread. Discard the centers.
3. Place the bread pieces in the butter in the pan.
4. Carefully crack an egg into the hole of each piece of bread.
5. Cook until the bread crisps and the egg whites set, about 3 minutes.
6. Flip and cook just until the yolk is almost set, 1 to 2 minutes more.

7. Season to taste with the salt and pepper.

Nutrition facts: Per Serving calories: 241 | fat: 17g | protein: 10g | carbs: 12g | sugars: 0g | fiber: 2g | sodium: 307mg

Walnut and Oat Granola

Prep time: 10 minutes

Cook time: 30 minutes

Serves: 16

Ingredients:

- 4 cups rolled oats
- 1 cup walnut pieces
- ½ cup pepitas
- ¼ teaspoon salt
- 1 teaspoon ground cinnamon
- 1 teaspoon ground ginger
- ½ cup coconut oil, melted
- ½ cup unsweetened applesauce
- 1 teaspoon vanilla extract
- ½ cup dried cherries

Instruction :

1. Preheat the oven to 350°F (180°C).
2. Line a baking sheet with parchment paper.
3. In a large bowl, toss the oats, walnuts, pepitas, salt, cinnamon, and ginger.
4. In a large measuring cup, combine the coconut oil, applesauce, and vanilla.
5. Pour over the dry mixture and mix well.
6. Transfer the mixture to the prepared baking sheet.
7. Cook for 30 minutes, stirring about halfway through.
8. Remove from the oven and let the granola sit undisturbed until completely cool.
9. Break the granola into pieces, and stir in the dried cherries.
10. Transfer to an airtight container, and store at room temperature for up to 2 weeks.

Nutrition facts: per Serving: calories: 225 fat: 14.9g protein: 4.9g carbs: 20.1g fiber: 3.1g sugar: 4.9g sodium: 31mg

Apple and Bran Muffins

Prep time: 10 minutes
Cook time: 20 minutes
Serves: 18 muffins
Ingredients:

- 2 cups whole-wheat flour
- 1 cup wheat bran
- 1/3 cup granulated sweetener
- 1 tablespoon baking powder
- 2 teaspoons ground cinnamon
- ½ teaspoon ground ginger
- ¼ teaspoon ground nutmeg Pinch sea salt
- 2 eggs
- 1½ cups skim milk, at room temperature
- ½ cup melted coconut oil
- 2 teaspoons pure vanilla extract 2
- apples, peeled, cored, and diced

Instructions:

1. Preheat the oven to 350°F (180°C).
2. Line 18 muffin cups with paper liners and set the tray aside.
3. In a large bowl, stir together the flour, bran, sweetener, baking powder, cinnamon, ginger, nutmeg, and salt.
4. In a small bowl, whisk the eggs, milk, coconut oil, and vanilla until blended.
5. Add the wet ingredients to the dry ingredients, stirring until just blended.
6. Stir in the apples and spoon equal amounts of batter into each muffin cup.
7. Bake the muffins until a toothpick inserted in the center of a muffin comes out clean, about 20 minutes.
8. Cool the muffins completely and serve.
9. Store leftover muffins in a sealed container in the refrigerator for up to 3 days or in the freezer for up to 1 month.

Nutrition facts: per Serving: calories: 142 fat: 7.1g protein: 4.1g carbs: 19.1g fiber: 3.1g sugar: 6.1g sodium: 21mg

Greek Yogurt and Oat Pancakes

Prep time: 5 minutes

Cook time: 20 minutes

Serves: 4

Ingredients:

- 1 cup 2 percent plain Greek yogurt
- 3 eggs
- 1½ teaspoons pure vanilla extract
- 1 cup rolled oats
- 1 tablespoon granulated sweetener
- 1 teaspoon baking powder
- 1 teaspoon ground cinnamon
  Pinch ground cloves
- Nonstick cooking spray

Instruction:

1. Place the yogurt, eggs, and vanilla in a blender and pulse to combine.
2. Add the oats, sweetener, baking powder, cinnamon, and cloves to the blender and blend until the batter is smooth.
3. Place a large nonstick skillet over medium heat and lightly coat it with cooking spray.
4. Spoon ¼ cup of batter per pancake, 4 at a time, into the skillet.
5. Cook the pancakes until the bottoms are firm and golden, about 4 minutes.
6. Flip the pancakes over and cook the other side until they are cooked through, about 3 minutes.
7. Remove the pancakes to a plate and repeat with the remaining batter.
8. Serve with fresh fruit.

Nutrition facts: per Serving: calories: 244 fat: 8.1g protein: 13.1g carbs: 28.1g fiber: 4.0g sugar: 3.0g sodium: 82mg

Asparagus Frittata

Prep time: 12 minutes

Cook time: 45 minutes

Serves: 6

Ingredients:

- 1 lb. of thin asparagus
- 2 onions, chopped
- 1 ½ teaspoons extra-virgin olive oil
- 1 red bell pepper, chopped
- 2 cloves garlic, minced
- ½ cup of water
- 4 large eggs
- 2 large egg whites
- 1 cup part-skim ricotta cheese
- ½ teaspoon sea salt, divided
- 1 tablespoon parsley, fresh chopped
- ½ cup Gruyere cheese, shredded
- 2 tablespoons breadcrumbs, dry

Instructions:

1. Preheat your oven to 325° Fahrenheit.
2. Coat a 10-inch pie pan with some cooking spray.
3. Sprinkle pan with breadcrumbs.
4. Remove the tough ends of the asparagus: slice tips off and reserve.
5. Slice the asparagus stalks into 1/2-inch-long slices.
6. Heat your oil in a nonstick pan over medium-high heat.
7. Next, add the bell pepper, onions, garlic and ¼ teaspoon sea salt.
8. Cook for 7 minutes.
9. Add water to the asparagus stalks in the pan and cook while stirring until asparagus is tender, for about 7 minutes or until the liquid is evaporated.
10. Season with salt and pepper as needed, arranging the vegetables in an even layer in the pan.
11. Whisk your egg whites and eggs in a mixing bowl.
12. Add the ricotta, parsley and remaining sea salt and pepper, then whisk to blend.
13. Pour your egg mixture over the vegetables in the pan while gently shaking the pan to distribute evenly.

14. Scatter your reserved asparagus tips over the top along with the Gruyere.
15. Bake your frittata until a knife inserted in the middle comes out clean.
16. It should take about 35 minutes.
17. Let your frittata stand for about 5 minutes before serving.
18. Serve and enjoy!

Nutrition facts: (per 1/6 of recipe): Calories: 193 Fat: 11g Protein: 15g Carbs: 10g

Whole-Grain Dutch Baby Pancake

Prep Time: 5 minutes

Cook Time: 25 minutes

Serves: 4

Ingredients:

- 2 tablespoons coconut oil
- 1/2 cup whole-wheat flour
- ¼ cup skim milk
- 3 large eggs
- 1 teaspoon vanilla extract
- 1/2 teaspoon baking powder
- ¼ teaspoon salt
- ¼ teaspoon ground cinnamon
- Powdered sugar, for dusting

Instructions:

1. Preheat the oven to 400f.
2. Put the coconut oil in a medium oven-safe skillet, and place the skillet in the oven to melt the oil while it preheats.
3. In a blender, combine the flour, milk, eggs, vanilla, baking powder, salt, and cinnamon.
4. Process until smooth.
5. Carefully remove the skillet from the oven and tilt to spread the oil around evenly.
6. Pour the batter into the skillet and return it to the oven for 23 to 25 minutes, until the pancake puffs and lightly browns.
7. Remove, dust lightly with powdered sugar, cut into 4 wedges, and serve.

Nutrition Facts: Calories: 195; Total Fat: 11g; Saturated Fat: 7g; Protein: 8g; Carbs: 16g; Sugar: 1g; Fiber: 2g; Cholesterol: 140mg; Sodium: 209mg

Lovely Porridge

Prep Time: 15 minutes

Cook Time: Nil

Serves: 2

Ingredients:

- 2 tablespoons coconut flour
- 2 tablespoons vanilla protein powder
- 3 tablespoons Golden Flaxseed meal
- 1 and 1/2 cups almond milk, unsweetened
- Powdered erythritol

Instructions:

1. Take a bowl and mix in flaxseed meal, protein powder, coconut flour and mix well
2. Add mix to the saucepan (placed over medium heat)
3. Add almond milk and stir, let the mixture thicken
4. Add your desired amount of sweetener and serve
5. Enjoy!

Nutrition facts: Calories: 259; Fat: 13g; Carbohydrates: 5g; Protein: 16g

Greek Chicken Breast

Prep Time: 10 minutes
Cook Time: 25 minutes
Serves: 4
Ingredients:

- 4 chicken breast halves, skinless and boneless
- 1 cup extra virgin olive oil
- 1 lemon, juiced

- 2 teaspoons garlic, crushed
- 1 and 1/2 teaspoons black pepper
- 1/3 teaspoon paprika

Instructions:

1. Cut 3 slits in the chicken breast
2. Take a small bowl and whisk in olive oil, salt, lemon juice, garlic, paprika, pepper and whisk for 30 seconds
3. Place chicken in a large bowl and pour marinade
4. Rub the marinade all over using your hand Refrigerate overnight
5. Pre-heat grill to medium heat and oil the grate
6. Cook chicken in the grill until center is no longer pink
7. Serve and enjoy!

Nutrition facts: Calories: 644; Fat: 57g; Carbohydrates: 2g; Protein: 27g

Breakfast Salad

Prep Time: 5 minutes

Cook Time: 15 minutes

Serves: 3

Ingredients:

- 1 cup finely diced kale
- 1 cup cabbage, red and Chinese
- 2 tbsp. coconut oil
- 1 cup spinach
- 2 moderate avocados
- 1.2kg chickpeas sprout
- 2 tbsp. sunflower seed sprouts
- Pure sea salt (seasoning)
- Bell pepper (seasoning)
- Lemon juice (seasoning)

Instructions:

1. Add spinach, Chinese and red cabbage, kale, coconut oil, to a container.
2. Add seasoning to taste and mix adequately.
3. Add other ingredients and mix.

Nutrition facts: Calories: 112 Protein: 28g Fiber: 10g Sugar: 1g

Cheese Yogurt

Prep Time: 12 minutes

Cook Time: 15 minutes

Serves: 2

Ingredients:

- 1 thick and Creamy Yogurt or store-bought yogurt
- ½ tsp. kosher salt

Instructions:

1. Line a strainer of twice the normal or plastic cheesecloth thickness.
2. Place the strainer on top of a bowl and apply the yogurt.
3. Cover and refrigerate for 2 hours.
4. Stir in the salt and continue to drip for another 2 hours until the yogurt cheese is ready to spread.

Nutrition facts: Calories: 83 Protein: 5g Fat: 5.4g

Breakfast Cake

Prep time: 5 minutes

Cook time: 45 minutes

Serves: 4

Ingredients:

- Coconut flour, 1/2 cup
- Vanilla protein powder, 3-4 tablespoons
- Baking soda, 1/2 teaspoon
- Salt, 1/8 teaspoon
- Eggs, 6
- Olive oil, 1/4 cup
- Water, 3/4 cup
- Baking paper

Instructions:

1. Preheat your oven to 350°Fahrenheit/180°Celsius.
2. Inside a food processor, mix the first 4 items for 10 seconds.
3. Toss in the remaining ingredients until well mixed.
4. Line the lower end and edges of a squared baking tray (20cm/ 8") using baking paper, now pour the

flour mixture within the frying pan.
5. Cook for around 60-50 minutes, then remove from oven, allow to cool before serving.

Nutritional Facts: Fat: 12g, Net Carbs: 6g, Protein: 15g, Sodium: 18mg

Lunch

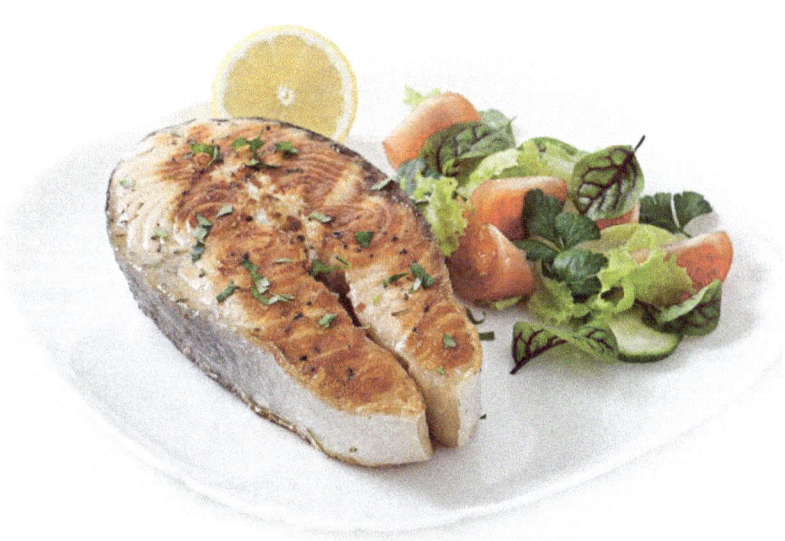

Brunswick Stew

Prep Time: 10 minutes
Cook Time: 45 minutes
Serves: 3
Ingredients:
- 4 ounces diced salt pork
- 2 pounds chicken parts
- 8 cups water
- 3 potatoes, cubed
- 3 onions, chopped
- 1 (28 ounce) can whole peeled tomatoes
- 2 cups canned whole kernel corn
- 1 (10 ounce) package frozen lima beans
- 1 tablespoon Worcestershire sauce
- 1/2 teaspoon salt
- 1/4 teaspoon ground black pepper

Instructions:
1. Mix and boil water, chicken and salt pork in a big pot on high heat. Lower heat to low. Cover then simmer until chicken is tender for 45 minutes.
2. Take out chicken. Let cool until easily handled.
3. Take meat out. Throw out bones and skin.
4. Chop meat to bite-sized pieces.
5. Put back in the soup.
6. Add ground black pepper, salt, Worcestershire sauce, lima beans, corn, tomatoes, onions and potatoes.
7. Mix well. Stir well and simmer for 1 hour, uncovered.

Nutrition facts: 368 Calories; 25.9g Carbohydrate; 27.9g Protein

Chicken Chili

Prep Time: 6 minutes
Cook Time: 1 hour
Serves: 4
Ingredients:

- 3 tablespoons vegetable oil
- 2 cloves garlic, minced
- 1 green bell pepper, chopped
- 1 onion, chopped
- 1 stalk celery, sliced
- 1/4-pound mushrooms, chopped
- 1-pound chicken breast
- 1 tablespoon chili powder
- 1 teaspoon dried oregano
- 1 teaspoon ground cumin
- 1/2 teaspoon paprika
- 1/2 teaspoon cocoa powder
- 1/4 teaspoon salt
- 1 pinch crushed red pepper flakes
- 1 pinch ground black pepper
- 1 (14.5 oz) can tomatoes with juice
- 1 (19 oz) can kidney beans

Instructions:

1. Fill 2 tablespoons of oil into a big skillet and heat it at moderate heat.
2. Add mushrooms, celery, onion, bell pepper and garlic, sautéing for 5 minutes.
3. Put it to one side.
4. Insert the leftover 1 tablespoon of oil into the skillet.
5. At high heat, cook the chicken until browned and its exterior turns firm.
6. Transfer the vegetable mixture back into skillet.
7. Stir in ground black pepper, hot pepper flakes, salt, cocoa powder, paprika, oregano, cumin and chili powder.
8. Continue stirring for several minutes to avoid burning.
9. Pour in the beans and tomatoes and lead the entire mixture to boiling point then adjust the setting to low heat.
10. Place a lid on the skillet and leave it simmering for 15 minutes.
11. Uncover the skillet and leave it simmering for another 15 minutes.

Nutrition facts: 308 Calories; 25.9g Carbohydrate; 29g Protein

Chicken and Pepperoni

Prep Time: 4 minutes
Cook Time: 4 hours
Serves: 5

Ingredients:
- 3½ to 4 pounds meaty chicken pieces
- 1/8 teaspoon salt
- 1/8 teaspoon black pepper
- 2 ounces sliced turkey pepperoni
- ¼ cup sliced pitted ripe olives
- ½ cup reduced-sodium chicken broth
- 1 tablespoon tomato paste
- 1 teaspoon dried Italian seasoning, crushed
- ½ cup shredded part-skim mozzarella cheese (2 ounces)

Instructions:
1. Put chicken into a 3 1/2 to 5-qt. slow cooker.
2. Sprinkle pepper and salt on the chicken.
3. Slice pepperoni slices in half.
4. Put olives and pepperoni into the slow cooker.
5. In a small bowl, blend Italian seasoning, tomato paste and chicken broth together.
6. Transfer the mixture into the slow cooker.
7. Cook with a cover for 3-3 1/2 hours on high.
8. Transfer the olives, pepperoni and chicken onto a serving platter with a slotted spoon.
9. Discard the cooking liquid.
10. Sprinkle cheese over the chicken.
11. Use foil to loosely cover and allow to sit for 5 minutes to melt the cheese.

Nutrition facts: 243 Calories; 1g Carbohydrate; 41g Protein

Comforting Summer Squash Soup with Crispy Chickpeas

Prep Time: 10 minutes
Cook Time: 20 minutes
Serves: 4
Ingredients:

- 1 (15-ounce) can low-sodium chickpeas
- 1 teaspoon extra-virgin olive oil
- ¼ teaspoon smoked paprika
- Pinch salt, plus
- ½ teaspoon
- 3 medium zucchinis
- 3 cups low-sodium vegetable broth
- ½ onion
- 3 garlic cloves
- 2 tablespoons plain low-fat Greek yogurt Freshly ground black pepper

Instructions:

1. Preheat the oven to 425°F.
2. Line a baking sheet with parchment paper.
3. In a medium mixing bowl, toss the chickpeas with 1 teaspoon of olive oil, the smoked paprika, and a pinch salt.
4. Transfer to the prepared baking sheet and roast until crispy, about 20 minutes, stirring once.
5. Set aside.
6. Meanwhile, in a medium pot, heat the remaining 1 tablespoon of oil over medium heat.
7. Add the zucchini, broth, onion, and garlic to the pot, and boil.
8. Simmer, and cook for 20 minutes.
9. In a blender jar, purée the soup.
10. Return to the pot.
11. Add the yogurt, remaining ½ teaspoon of salt, and pepper, and stir well.
12. Serve topped with the roasted chickpeas.

Nutrition facts: 188 Calories; 24g Carbohydrates; 7g Sugars

Arugula and Avocado Salad

Prep time: 5 min
Cook time: 15-20 minutes
Serves: 4
Ingredients:
- 1 bunch arugula leaves
- 2 avocados, peeled and sliced
- 1 cup strawberries, halved
- 1/2 cup corn kernels, cooked
- 1 tbsp poppy seeds
- 1 tbsp lemon juice
- 2 tbsp extra virgin olive oil

Instructions:
1. Combine all ingredients in a salad bowl and gently toss.
2. Sprinkle with lemon juice and olive oil, stir, top with poppy seeds and serve.

Nutrition facts: calories: 226 fat: 19.05g protein: 3.16g carbs: 15.31g fiber: 8.4g sodium:

Bean and Scallion Salad

Prep Time: 10 minutes
Cook Time: 0 minute
Serves: 8
Ingredients:
- 1 (15 oz.) can low-sodium chickpeas
- 1 (15 oz.) can low-sodium kidney beans
- 1 (15 oz.) can low-sodium white beans
- 1 red bell pepper
- ¼ cup chopped scallions
- ¼ cup finely chopped fresh basil
- 3 garlic cloves, minced
- 2 tbsp. extra-virgin olive oil
- 1 tbsp. red wine vinegar
- 1 tsp. Dijon mustard
- ¼ tsp. freshly ground black pepper

Instruction:
1. Toss chickpeas, kidney beans, white beans, bell pepper, scallions, basil, and garlic gently.
2. Blend together olive oil, vinegar, mustard, and pepper.

3. Toss with the salad.
4. Wrap and chill for 1 hour.

Nutrition facts: Calories: 193
Carbohydrates: 29g Sugar: 3g

Chicken Vera Cruz

Prep Time: 7 minutes
Cook Time: 10 hours
Servings: 5
Ingredients:
- 1 medium onion, cut into wedges
- 1 lb. yellow-skin potatoes
- 6 skinless, boneless chicken thighs
- 2 (14.5 oz.) cans no-salt-added diced tomatoes
- 1 fresh jalapeño chili pepper
- 2 tbsp. Worcestershire sauce
- 1 tbsp. chopped garlic
- 1 tsp. dried oregano, crushed
- ¼ tsp. ground cinnamon
- ⅛ tsp. ground cloves
- ½ cup snipped fresh parsley
- ¼ cup chopped pimiento-stuffed green olives

Instruction:
1. Put the onion in a 3 ½ or 4-quart slow cooker.
2. Place chicken thighs and potatoes on top.
3. Drain and discard juices from a can of tomatoes.
4. Stir undrained and drained tomatoes, cloves, cinnamon, oregano, garlic, Worcestershire sauce, and jalapeño pepper together in a bowl.
5. Pour over all in the cooker.
6. Cook with a cover for 10 hours on a low-heat setting.
7. To make the topping: Stir chopped pimiento-stuffed green olives and snipped fresh parsley together in a small bowl.
8. Drizzle the topping over each serving of chicken.

Nutrition facts: Calories: 228 Sugar: 9g Carbohydrate: 25g

Fire-Roasted Tomatoes Over Chicken

Prep time: 10 minutes
Cook time: 20 minutes
Serving: 2
Ingredients:
- Garlic-herb blend,
- 2.5 tablespoons Salt,
- 1/2 teaspoon Italian seasoning,
- 1-1/4 teaspoon Pepper,
- 1/4 teaspoon Red pepper flakes,
- 1/8 teaspoon (optional) Debone chicken breast,
- 4 Olive oil,
- 1-2 tablespoons Chopped tomatoes,
- 1 can Chopped green beans,
- 3/4 pound Water,
- 2 tablespoons Butter,
- 1 tablespoon Cooked pasta, optional

Instructions.
1. Combine the seasoning ingredients and sprinkle on all the sides of the chicken breasts.
2. Warm the oil inside a big pan on a medium flame.
3. Brown all sides of the chicken.
4. Add chopped tomatoes and bring to a simmer.
5. Reduce heat to low and cover for 11-13 minutes, otherwise until a digital thermometer inserted into the chicken reaches 165°.
6. Meanwhile, mix green beans and tomatoes with water inside a 2-quart oven-safe dish; microwave on high temperature for 5-6 minutes, until it's tender.
7. Drain.
8. Now remove the chicken from the pan; keep warm.
9. Whisk in the butter and chopped beans into the prepared tomato mixture.
10. End up serving with chicken and cooked pasta, if needed.

Nutritional Facts: Fat: 10g, Net Carbs: 12g, Protein: 37g, Sodium: 681mg

Vegetable Minestrone Soup

Prep time: 30 minutes
Cook time: 360 minutes
Serving: 8
Ingredients:
1. 1/2 cup Diced carrots,
2. 4 Celery stalks, diced,
3. 3 Diced red onion,
4. 1 Chopped garlic cloves,
5. 3 Green beans flaked,
6. 2-1/2 cups Red kidney beans,
7. 15 ounces Tomatoes, undrained,
8. 15 ounces Vegetable broth,
9. 6-1/2 cups Italian seasoning,
10. 2 tablespoons Red pepper,
11. 1 teaspoon Salt,
12. 3/4 teaspoon Pepper,
13. 1/2 teaspoon Diced zucchini,
14. 1 Elbow pasta,
15. 4 ounces Parmesan cheese,

Instructions:
1. Combine the first 12 ingredients inside a 6- to 8-quart slow cooker.
2. Cook on low flame for 7 to 8 hours, covered.
3. Whisk in the zucchini, followed by pasta, and season with salt.
4. Cover, and Cook, on low flame for 16 to 22 minutes more, otherwise until the pasta becomes soft.
5. Serve cheese on top.
6. Have fun!

Nutrition Facts Fat: 2g, Net Carbs: 41g, Protein: 11g, Sodium: 525mg

Three-Pepper Pizza

Prep time: 10 minutes
Cook time: 15 minutes
Serving: 4
Ingredients:
- 1/2 Italian seasoning,
- 1/4 teaspoon Tomato paste,
- 1/3 cup Water,
- 1/4 cup Pizza crust,
- 1 (12-inch) Mozzarella cheese,
- 1 cup Red bell pepper,
- 1 1/2 cups Onion, chopped,

Instructions:
1. Preheat the oven to 450F.
2. In a medium mixing cup, combine the seasoning, some tomato paste with water; stir well.
3. Spread on top of pizza crust.
4. Sprinkle the cheese on top.
5. Sprinkle the bell pepper and the onion evenly over the cheese.
6. Bake for about 10 to 12 mins, or until the cheese melts, at about 450°.
7. Cut into the 6 wedges and serve.

Nutritional Facts Fat: 2g, Net Carbs: 36g, Protein: 10g, Sodium: 352mg

Parmesan Baked Cod

Prep time: 5 minutes
Cook time: 20 minutes
Serving: 4
Ingredients:
- Cod fillets, 4
- Parmesan cheese, 1/4 cup
- Worcestershire sauce, 1 teaspoon
- Mayonnaise, 2/3 cup
- Chopped green onions, 4

Instructions:
1. Preheat your oven to 375 degrees Fahrenheit.
2. Place the cod in an 8-inch square shape baking dish that has been sprayed with nonstick cooking spray.
3. Combine the remaining ingredients and scatter them over the fillets.
4. Finally, Bake the fillets for 10-15 minutes, or until they start to flake nicely with a fork.
5. Serve with lemon wedges, and enjoy!

Nutritional Facts Fat: 15g, Net Carbs: 7g, Protein: 20g, Sodium: 450mg

Cilantro Lime Shrimp

Prep time: 10 minutes
Cook time: 20 minutes
Serving: 4
Ingredients:
1. Fresh cilantro, 1/3 cup
2. Lime zest, 1-1/2 teaspoons
3. Minced garlic cloves, 3
4. Salt, 1/4 teaspoon
5. Ground cumin, 1/4 teaspoon
6. Pepper, 1/4 teaspoon
7. Uncooked shrimp, 1 pound
8. Lime slices, 3-4
9. Lime juice, 1/3 cup
10. Jalapeno pepper, 1
11. Olive oil, 2 tablespoons

Instructions:
1. Toss the shrimp with the first nine ingredients.
2. Allow resting for 15 minutes.
3. Thread the shrimps over metal or water-soaked wooden skewers, then thread some lime slices as well.
4. Cover and grill the skewers over medium heat for 3-5 minutes per side before the shrimp turn yellow.
5. Serve and enjoy!

Nutritional Facts Fat: 8g, Net Carbs: 4g, Protein: 19g, Sodium: 284mg
Nutritional Facts Fat: 22g, Net Carbs: 17g, Protein: 28g, Sodium:

Turkey Coriander Dish

Prep Time: 20 minutes
Cook Time: 20 minutes
Serves: 4
Ingredients:
- Half bunch coriander (sliced)
- 1 cup chard (sliced)
- 1 piece (no bones and skin) turkey breast
- 1 and a half cup coconut cream
- 2 pieces garlic cloves
- 1 tbsp. melted ghee

Instructions:
1. Put the instant pot on the "Sauté" option, then put the ghee and cook it.
2. After that, put the garlic and meat, then heat it for 5 minutes.
3. Put the other ingredients, then cover it and heat it for 25 minutes at a high temperature.
4. Release the pressure gradually for 10 minutes, then split them among your plates before eating.

Nutrition facts: Calories: 225 Fat: 8.9 g Fiber: 0.2 g Carbs: 0.8 g Protein: 33.5 g

Lentil And Eggplant Stew

Prep time: 10 minutes
Cook time: 30 minutes
Serves: 2
Ingredients:
- 1 lb. eggplant
- 1 lb. dry lentils
- 1 cup chopped vegetables
- 1 cup low sodium vegetable broth

Instructions:
1. Mix all the ingredients in your Instant Pot, cook on Stew for 35 minutes.
2. Release the pressure naturally and serve.

Nutrition facts: Calories 310, Carbs 22g, Fat 10g, Protein 32g, Potassium (K) 670.6 mg, Sodium (Na) 267 mg

Eggplant Curry

Prep time: 10 minutes

Cook time: 30 minutes

Serves: 2

Ingredients:

- 2-3 cups chopped eggplant
- 1 thinly sliced onion
- 1 cup coconut milk
- 3tbsp curry paste
- 1tbsp oil or ghee

Instructions:

1. Set the Instant Pot to saute and add the onion, oil, and curry paste.
2. When the onion is soft, add the remaining ingredients and seal.
3. Cook on Stew for 20 minutes.
4. Release the pressure naturally.

Nutrition facts: Calories: 350; Carbs: 15 ;Sugar: 3 ;Fat: 25 ;Protein: 11 ;GL

Blueberry and Chicken Salad

Prep Time: 10 minutes

Cook Time: 0 minute

Serves: 4

Ingredients:

- 2 cups chopped cooked chicken
- 1 cup fresh blueberries
- ¼ cup almonds
- 1 celery stalk
- ¼ cup red onion
- 1 tablespoon fresh basil
- 1 tablespoon fresh cilantro
- ½ cup plain, vegan mayonnaise
- ¼ teaspoon salt
- ¼ teaspoon freshly ground black pepper
- 8 cups salad greens

Instructions:

1. Toss chicken, blueberries, almonds, celery, onion, basil, and cilantro.
2. Blend yogurt, salt, and pepper.
3. Stir chicken salad to combine.
4. Situate 2 cups of salad greens on each of 4 plates and divide the

chicken salad among the plates to serve.

Nutrition facts: 207 Calories; 11g Carbohydrates; 6g Sugars

Buffalo Chicken Salads

Prep Time: 7 minutes

Cook Time: 3 hours

Serves: 5

Ingredients:

- 1½ pounds chicken breast halves
- ½ cup Wing Time® Buffalo chicken sauce
- 4 teaspoons cider vinegar
- 1 teaspoon Worcestershire sauce
- 1 teaspoon paprika
- 1/3 cup light mayonnaise
- 2 tablespoons fat-free milk
- 2 tablespoons crumbled blue cheese
- 2 romaine hearts, chopped
- 1 cup whole grain croutons
- ½ cup very thinly sliced red onion

Instructions:

1. Place chicken in a 2-quarts slow cooker.
2. Mix together Worcestershire sauce, 2 teaspoons of vinegar and Buffalo sauce in a small bowl; pour over chicken.
3. Dust with paprika.
4. Close and cook for 3 hours on low-heat setting.
5. Mix the leftover 2 teaspoons of vinegar with milk and light mayonnaise together in a small bowl at serving time; mix in blue cheese.
6. While chicken is still in the slow cooker, pull meat into bite-sized pieces using two forks.
7. Split the romaine among 6 dishes.
8. Spoon sauce and chicken over lettuce.
9. Pour with blue cheese dressing then add red onion slices and croutons on top.

Nutrition facts: 274 Calories; 11g Carbohydrate; 2g Fiber

Chicken and Cornmeal Dumplings

Prep Time: 8 minutes

Cook Time: 8 hours

Serves: 4

Ingredients:

- Chicken and Vegetable Filling
- 2 medium carrots, thinly sliced
- 1 stalk celery, thinly sliced
- 1/3 cup corn kernels
- ½ of a medium onion, thinly sliced
- 2 cloves garlic, minced
- 1 teaspoon snipped fresh rosemary
- ¼ teaspoon ground black pepper
- 2 chicken thighs, skinned
- 1 cup reduced sodium chicken broth
- ½ cup fat-free milk
- 1 tablespoon all-purpose flour
  Cornmeal Dumplings
- ¼ cup flour
- ¼ cup cornmeal
- ½ teaspoon baking powder
- 1 egg white
- 1 tablespoon fat-free milk
- 1 tablespoon canola oil

Instructions:

1. Mix 1/4 teaspoon pepper, carrots, garlic, celery, rosemary, corn, and onion in a 1 1/2 or 2-quart slow cooker.
2. Place chicken on top.
3. Pour the broth atop mixture in the cooker.
4. Close and cook on low-heat for 7 to 8 hours.

5. If cooking with the low-heat setting, switch to high-heat setting (or if heat setting is not available, continue to cook).
6. Place the chicken onto a cutting board and let to cool slightly.
7. Once cool enough to handle, chop off chicken from bones and get rid of the bones.
8. Chop the chicken and place back into the mixture in cooker.
9. Mix flour and milk in a small bowl until smooth.
10. Stir into the mixture in cooker.
11. Drop the Cornmeal Dumplings dough into 4 mounds atop hot chicken mixture using two spoons.
12. Cover and cook for 20 to 25 minutes more or until a toothpick come out clean when inserted into a dumpling. (Avoid lifting lid when cooking.)
13. Sprinkle each of the serving with coarse pepper if desired.
14. Mix together 1/2 teaspoon baking powder, 1/4 cup flour, a dash of salt and 1/4 cup cornmeal in a medium bowl.
15. Mix 1 tablespoon canola oil, 1 egg white and 1 tablespoon fat-free milk in a small bowl.
16. Pour the egg mixture into the flour mixture.
17. Mix just until moistened.

Nutrition facts: 369 Calories; 9g Sugar; 47g Carbohydrate

Moroccan Eggplant Stew

Prep time: 20 minutes
Cook time: 3 minutes
Serves: 4
Ingredients
- 2 tablespoons avocado oil
- 1 large onion, minced
- 2 garlic cloves, minced
- 1 teaspoon ras el hanout spice blend or curry powder

- ¼ teaspoon cayenne pepper
- 1 teaspoon kosher salt
- 1 cup vegetable broth or water
- 1 tablespoon tomato paste
- 2 cups chopped eggplant
- 2 medium gold potatoes, peeled and chopped
- 4 ounces (113 g) tomatillos, husks removed, chopped
- 1 (14-ounce / 397-g) can diced tomatoes

Instruction:

1. Set the electric pressure cooker to the Sauté setting.
2. When the pot is hot, pour in the avocado oil.
3. Sauté the onion for 3 to 5 minutes, until it begins to soften.
4. Add the garlic, ras el hanout, cayenne, and salt.
5. Cook and stir for about 30 seconds.
6. Hit Cancel.
7. Stir in the broth and tomato paste.
8. Add the eggplant, potatoes, tomatillos, and tomatoes with their juices.
9. Close and lock the lid of the pressure cooker.
10. Set the valve to sealing.
11. Cook on high pressure for 3 minutes.
12. When the cooking is complete, hit Cancel and allow the pressure to release naturally.
13. Once the pin drops, unlock and remove the lid.
14. Stir well and spoon into serving bowls.

Nutrition facts: per, Serving (1½ cups) calories: 216 fats: 8g protein: 4g carbs: 28g sugars: 9g fiber: 8g sodium:

Crispy Dill Salmon

Prep Time: 05 min
Cook Time: 15 min
Serves: 4

Ingredients

- 1 cup panko bread crumbs
- 2 tablespoons olive oil
- 2 tablespoons snipped fresh dill
- 1/4 teaspoon salt
- 1/8 teaspoon pepper
- 4 Salmon fillets (6 ounces each)
- 1 tablespoon lemon juice Lemon wedges

Instruction:

1. Preheat the oven to 400 °.
2. Mix the first 5 ingredients.
3. Place the salmon in a 15 x 10 x 1-inch container.
4. Baking dish covered with cooking spray; Brush with lemon juice.
5. Top with breadcrumb mixture, pat to stick.
6. Bake uncovered on an upper rack of the oven until fish flakes easily with a fork, 12 to 15 minutes.
7. Serve with lemon wedges.

Nutrition facts: Calories 408 Total Fat 19.5g25% Saturated Fat 2.9g15%Cholesterol 78mg26% Sodium 427mg19% Total Carbohydrate 20.6g7% Dietary Fiber 1.5g5% Total Sugars 1.8g Protein 38.5g

Green Salad with Berries and Sweet Potatoes

Prep Time: 15 minutes
Cook Time: 20 minutes
Serves: 4
Ingredients:
For the vinaigrette:
- 1-pint blackberries
- 2 tbsp. red wine vinegar
- 1 tbsp. honey
- 3 tbsp. extra-virgin olive oil
- ¼ tsp. salt Freshly ground black pepper

For The Salad:
- 1 sweet potato, cubed
- 1 tsp. extra-virgin olive oil
- 8 cups salad greens (baby spinach, spicy greens, romaine)
- ½ red onion, sliced
- ¼ cup crumbled goat cheese

Instruction:
For The Vinaigrette:
1. In a blender jar, combine the blackberries, vinegar, honey, oil, salt, and pepper, and process until smooth.
2. Set aside.

For The Salad:
1. Preheat the oven to 425°F. Line a baking sheet with parchment paper.
2. Mix the sweet potato with the olive oil.
3. Transfer to the prepared baking sheet and roast for 20 minutes, stirring once halfway through, until tender.
4. Remove and cool for a few minutes.
5. In a large bowl, toss the greens with the red onion and cooled sweet potato, and drizzle with the vinaigrette.
6. Serve topped with 1 tbsp. goat cheese per serving.

Nutrition facts: Calories: 196 Carbohydrates: 21g Sugar: 10g

Blueberry and Chicken Salad

Nutrition facts: Calories: 207

Carbohydrates: 11g Sugar: 6g

Prep Time: 10 minutes

Cook Time: 0 minute

Serves: 4

Ingredients:

- 2 cups chopped cooked chicken
- 1 cup fresh blueberries
- ¼ cup almonds
- 1 celery stalk
- ¼ cup red onion
- 1 tbsp. fresh basil
- 1 tbsp. fresh cilantro
- ½ cup plain, vegan mayonnaise
- ¼ tsp. salt
- ¼ tsp. freshly ground black pepper
- 8 cups salad greens

Instruction:

1. Toss chicken, blueberries, almonds, celery, onion, basil, and cilantro.
2. Blend yogurt, salt, and pepper.
3. Stir chicken salad to combine.
4. Situate 2 cups of salad greens on each of 4 plates and divide the chicken salad among the plates to serve.

Buffalo Chicken Salads

Preparation Time: 7 minutes

Cooking Time: 3 hours

Servings: 5

Ingredients:

- 1½ pounds chicken breast halves
- ½ cup Wing Time® Buffalo chicken sauce
- 4 tsp. cider vinegar
- 1 tsp. Worcestershire sauce
- 1 tsp. paprika
- 1/3 cup light mayonnaise
- 2 tbsp. fat-free milk
- 2 tbsp. crumbled blue cheese
- 2 romaine hearts, chopped
- 1 cup whole-grain croutons
- ½ cup very thinly sliced red onion

Instruction:

1. Place chicken in a 2/4 slow cooker.

2. Mix together Worcestershire sauce, 2 tsp. of vinegar and Buffalo sauce in a small bowl; pour over chicken.
3. Dust with paprika.
4. Close and cook for 3 hours on a low-heat setting.
5. Mix the leftover 2 tsp. of vinegar with milk and light mayonnaise together in a small bowl at serving time; mix in blue cheese.
6. While chicken is still in the slow cooker, pull meat into bite-sized pieces using 2 forks.
7. Split the romaine among 6 dishes.
8. Spoon sauce and chicken over lettuce.
9. Pour with blue cheese dressing then add red onion slices and croutons on top.

Nutrition facts: Calories: 274 Carbohydrate: 11g Fiber: 2g

Orange Chicken Thighs

Prep time: 20 minutes
Cook time: 300 minutes
Serving: 4
Ingredients:
- Sliced fresh carrots,
- 2 cups Sliced tomatoes,
- 1 can Diced medium onion,
- 1 Tomato paste,
- 1 can Orange juice,
- 1-1/2 cup Chopped garlic cloves,
- 2 Dried basils,
- 2-3 teaspoons Sugar,
- 1-1/2 teaspoons Dried oregano,
- 1-1/2 teaspoon Dried thyme,
- 1-1/2 teaspoon Dried rosemary,
- 1-1/2 teaspoon Pepper,
- 1/2 teaspoon Grated orange zest,
- 2-3 teaspoons Debone chicken thighs,
- 8 Lemon juice,
- 2-3 tablespoons Baked bacon flakes, 4

Instructions:
1. Mix the first 12 items inside a 3-quart slow cooker.

2. Whisk in 1.5 teaspoon orange zest.
3. Now add the chicken on top and spoon the sauce over it.
4. Bake on low for 6-7 hours, or when the chicken is tender.
5. Transfer to a serving dish.
6. Add sauce over chicken thighs and whisk in 2-3 tablespoons lemon juice and leftover orange zest.
7. Scatter with bacon.
8. Then serve.

Nutrition Facts: 10g, Net Carbs: 15g, Protein: 25g, Sodium: 236mg

Artichoke Ratatouille Chicken

Prep time: 15 minutes
Cook time: 45 minutes
Serving: 4
Ingredients:
- Japanese eggplants,
- 3 Plum tomatoes,
- 4 Sweet yellow pepper,
- 1-2 Sweet red pepper,
- 1-2 Medium onion,
- 1 Quartered artichoke,
- 1 can Chopped thyme,
- 2-3 tablespoons Capers, drained,
- 2-3 tablespoons Olive oil,
- 2-3 tablespoons Chopped garlic cloves,
- 2 Creole seasoning,
- 1-2 teaspoons Debone chicken breasts,
- 1-1/2 pounds' White wine,
- 1 cup Grated Asiago cheese,
- 1-1/4 cup Cooked pasta, optional

Instructions:
1. Preheat the oven to 350°Fahrenheit.
2. Cut the eggplants, plum tomatoes, peppers, and medium onion into 3/4-inch pieces; transfer them to a big bowl.
3. Mix in artichoke hearts, chopped thyme, capers, oil, chopped garlic cloves, and 1.5 teaspoon Creole seasoning.
4. Garnish the chicken with the rest of the Creole seasoning.
5. Now spoon veggies mixture over chicken inside a 13x9-inch baking dish sprayed with cooking oil.
6. Drizzle the wine over the vegetables.
7. Cook for 30 minutes, protected.

8. Uncover and cook for another 35-45 minutes, or until the chicken is lightly browned and the vegetables are tender.
9. Garnish with grated cheese.
10. Serve with cooked pasta if desired.

Nutritional Facts: Fat: 9g, Net Carbs: 15g, Protein: 28g, Sodium: 438mg

Vegan Chili with White Bean

Prep time: 10 minutes
Cook time: 45 minutes
Serving: 4
Ingredients:

- 2.5 tablespoons Canola oil,
- 1/4 cup Diced Anaheim pepper,
- 2 cups Diced onion,
- 1 Chopped garlic cloves,
- 4 Quinoa, soaked,
- 1/2 cup Dried oregano,
- 4 teaspoons Ground cumin,
- 4 teaspoons Salt,
- 1 teaspoon Ground coriander,
- 1 teaspoon Ground pepper,
- 1 teaspoon Vegetable broth,
- 4 cups White beans,
- 15 ounces Chopped zucchini,
- 1 Diced cilantro,
- 1/4 cup Lime juice,

Instructions:

1. Heat oil inside a big pot on a medium flame.
2. Include the 1st 3 ingredients.
3. Cook, while constantly stirring, for 6 to 8 minutes, or until the veggies are tender.
4. Add quinoa, oregano, followed by cumin, salt, coriander, as well as pepper; cook them while stirring until fragrant, about 1 minute.
5. Whisk in the broth with beans.
6. Get the water to a boil.
7. Now reduce the flame and bring it to simmer.
8. Cook, moderately covered, for 20 minutes, while stirring occasionally.
9. Include zucchini; cover then cook, for 11 to 16 minutes or more, otherwise until the zucchini becomes tender and the chili has thickened.

10. Whisk in the cilantro with lime juice.
11. End up serving with lime wedges.

Nutrition Facts Fat: 11g, Net Carbs: 36g, Protein: 9g, Sodium: 529mg

Roasted Chickpea in Curry Bowl

Prep time: 15 minutes
Cook time: 45 minutes
Serving: 4
Ingredients:

- Olive oil, 2 tablespoons
- Curry powder, 1 tablespoon
- Salt, ½ teaspoon
- Head cauliflower, 1 medium
- Chickpeas, rinsed, 15 ounces
- Water, 1 ¼ cups
- Quinoa, rinsed, ⅔ cup
- Baby spinach, 4 cups
- Tahini, 2 tablespoons
- Lime juice, 1 teaspoon
- Clove Garlic, minced, 1
- Ground pepper, ⅛ teaspoon

Instructions:

1. Preheat the oven to 425°F.
2. Coat a large size baking sheet with the cooking spray.
3. In a medium-size mixing cup, combine the oil, some curry powder, and 1/2 teaspoon salt.
4. Toss in cauliflower and the chickpeas to coat.
5. Spread on prepared baking sheet.
6. Roast, stirring, for 20 mins, or till soft and brown.
7. Meanwhile, in a saucepan, add 1 1/4 cups of water, with quinoa and remaining 1/4 teaspoon salt.
8. Boil water over the medium-high flame.
9. Reduce heat to medium-low, cover, and cook for 12 to 15 mins, or till quinoa is tender.
10. Remove quinoa from heat and fluff with a fork.
11. Stir in the spinach, cover, and then allow to rest for 6 mins.
12. Meanwhile, in another bowl, combine tahini, 1 teaspoon lime zest, lime juice, 1 clove of garlic, pepper, and the remaining 2 tablespoons water.

13. Divide quinoa mixture into four dinner bowls.
14. Drizzle tahini dressing over cauliflower-chickpea mixture and serve to enjoy this recipe.

Nutritional Facts: Fat: 15g, Net Carbs: 43g, Protein: 13g, Sodium: 625mg

Pepper Steak Squash

Prep time: 10 minutes
Cook time: 30 minutes
Serving: 4
Ingredients:

- Beef broth, 1 can
- Soy sauce, 2.5 tablespoons
- Cornstarch, 3 tablespoons
- Canola oil, 2.5 tablespoons
- Beef flank steak, 1.5 pounds
- Green pepper, 1
- Sweet red pepper, about 1
- Zucchini, flaked, 2
- Onion, flaked, 1
- Garlic cloves, 3
- Snow peas, 1 cup
- Mushrooms, 1 cup
- Water chestnuts, 8.5 ounces
- Hot cooked rice, 1 bowl

Instructions:

1. Mix beef broth, soy sauce, including cornstarch inside a mixing bowl until smooth.
2. Place aside. Inside a big pan, warm 1 teaspoon oil over moderate flame.
3. Include beef and stir-fry for 3-4 minutes, or until the meat is properly cooked.
4. Take out from the skillet.
5. In the same pan, warm the remaining oil.
6. Include peppers and stir-fry for 2 minutes.
7. Include zucchini, onion with garlic; bake and stir for 2 minutes more.
8. Add snow peas and sliced mushrooms with water chestnuts.
9. Again, Stir-fry for 2 minutes, otherwise until crisp-tender.
10. Whisk cornstarch mixture, then add to skillet.

11. Now bring to a simmer while stirring until the sauce thickens, 1-2 minutes.
12. Transfer the meat to the pan; cook through.
13. End up serving with cooked rice.

Nutritional Facts Fat: 11g, Net Carbs: 16g, Protein: 18g, Sodium: 381mg

Flank Steak Beef

Prep Time: 10 minutes
Cook Time: 20 minutes
Serves: 4
Ingredients:
- 1-pound flank steaks, sliced
- ¼ cup xanthan gum
- 2 tsps. vegetable oil
- ½ tsp. ginger
- ½ cup soy sauce
- 1 tbsp. garlic, minced
- ½ cup water
- ¾ cup swerve, packed

Instructions:
1. Preheat the Air fryer to 390°F and grease an Air fryer basket.
2. Coat the steaks with xanthan gum on both sides and transfer them into the Air fryer basket.
3. Cook for about 10 minutes and dish out on a platter.
4. Meanwhile, cook the rest of the ingredients for the sauce in a saucepan.
5. Bring to a boil and pour over the steak slices to serve.

Nutrition facts: Calories: 372 Fat: 11.8 g Carbs: 1.8 g Sugar: 27.3 g Protein: 34 g Sodium: 871 mg

French Onion Soup

Prep time: 10 minutes

Cook time: 30 minutes

Serves: 2

Ingredients:

- 6 onions, chopped finely
- 2 cups vegetable broth
- 2tbsp oil
- 2tbsp Gruyere

Instructions:

1. Place the oil in your Instant Pot and cook the onions on Saute until soft and brown.
2. Mix all the ingredients in your Instant Pot.
3. Cook on Stew for 35 minutes.
4. Release the pressure naturally.

Nutrition facts: Calories: 110; Carbs: 8; Sugar: 3; Fat: 10; Protein: 3; GL: 4

Dinner

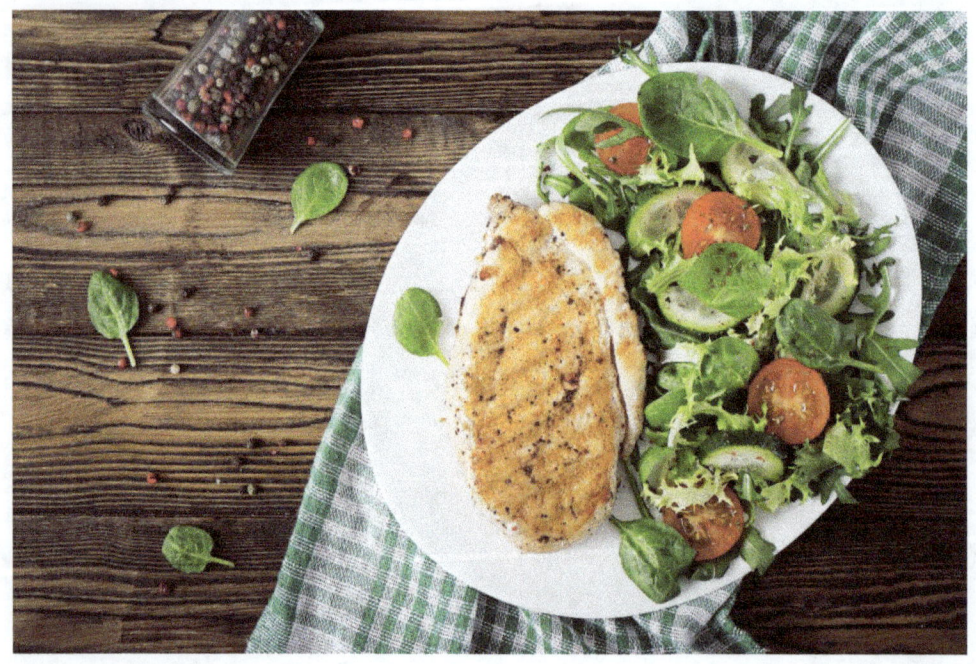

Herbed Chicken Meal

Prep Time: 5 minutes
Cook Time 25 minutes
Servings: 6

Ingredients
- cloves garlic
- 3 large boneless, skinless chicken breasts
- 3 tablespoons rosemary
- 3 tablespoons butter, melted
- 1½ tablespoons olive oil
- 1 teaspoon salt
- 1 cup dry vermouth
- ½ cup red wine vinegar
- ¾ teaspoon pink peppercorns

Directions
1. Divide the chicken breasts into halves and pat dry with paper towels.
2. Heat the butter and olive oil over medium heat in a medium saucepan or skillet.
3. Add the garlic and stir cook for 30 seconds until softened. Add the chicken breasts and stir-cook for 1–2 minutes until evenly brown.
4. Add the salt and vinegar; stir the mixture.
5. Cover and simmer over low heat for about 5 minutes.
6. Add the rosemary and vermouth; stir and simmer the mixture uncovered for about 10 minutes until the chicken is tender and well cooked.
7. Transfer the chicken to serving plates.
8. Add the peppercorns and simmer the mixture for 4–5 minutes.
9. Pour the mixture over the chicken and serve warm.

Nutrition facts: Calories 187 Fat 11.5 total carbs 1 sugar 0 g, Protein 16.5 sodium 183 mg

Italian Pork Chops

Prep Time: 5 minutes

Cook Time: 25 minutes

Servings: 4

Ingredients

- 4 cloves garlic, sliced 4 thick pork chops, fat trimmed
- 1 small yellow onion, cut into rings
- ½ cup low-fat mozzarella cheese
- 1 (28-ounce) can diced tomatoes
- 1 teaspoon paprika
- 1 teaspoon dried oregano
- 1 chicken bouillon cube Salt and pepper to taste

Directions

1. Preheat the oven to 400°F (200°C).
2. Grease a baking pan with some cooking spray.
3. Season the pork chops with pepper.
4. Grease a medium saucepan or skillet with cooking spray and heat it over medium heat.
5. Add the pork chops and stir-cook for 2 minutes per side until evenly brown.
6. Add the garlic and onion rings and stir-cook for 1–2 minutes until softened.
7. Add the spices, tomato and bouillon cube; simmer for 2–3 minutes. Pour in the tomato sauce.
8. Add the mixture to the baking pan, top with the cheese, and bake for about 20 minutes until the top is golden brown.
9. Let cool slightly and serve warm.
10. Note: You can store leftovers in an airtight container in the refrigerator for up to 3–4 days.
11. Simply reheat in a saucepan and serve.

Nutrition facts: Calories 405 Fat 17 g, Total carbs 16 g, Sugar 7.5 g, Protein 43.5 sodium 1275 mg

Baked Broccoli Chicken

Prep Time: 10 minutes

Cook Time 45 minutes

Servings: 4

Ingredients

- 1 teaspoon vegetable oil
- 4 medium chicken fillets, chopped
- 1 medium onion, finely chopped
- 1 (10.5-ounce) can chicken or mushroom soup
- 1-pound broccoli florets, boiled and drained
- 1 teaspoon curry powder
- 2 ounces' brown breadcrumbs
- 2 ounces' low-fat cheddar cheese, grated
- ½ cup skimmed milk Salt and pepper to taste

Directions

1. Preheat the oven to 425°F (220°C).
2. Grease a baking dish or casserole dish with some cooking spray.
3. Heat the oil over medium heat in a medium saucepan or skillet.
4. Add the onion and stir-cook until softened and translucent.
5. Add the chicken pieces; stir-cook for 10 minutes until evenly brown.
6. Set aside. Add the chicken or mushroom soup, milk and curry powder to a mixing bowl. Mix well.
7. Arrange the chicken mixture and broccoli in the baking dish; pour the soup mixture on top.
8. Top with the crumbs and cheddar cheese.
9. Bake for about 30 minutes until the top is evenly brown. Slice and serve warm.

Nutrition facts: Calories 332 Fat 9 g Total carbs 15 g Sugar 6 g, Protein 44.5 g Sodium 700 mg

Chicken breast on vegetable noodles

Prep Time: 10 minutes

Cook Time: 40 minutes

Servings: 4

Ingredients

- 300 g of chicken breast fillet
- Sea salt
- 1 organic zucchini, yellow (300 g)
- 1 organic zucchini, green (300 g)
- 200 g organic carrots
- 125 g chicory
- 1 tbsp. sesame oil 3 tbsp.& soy sauce, light, sugar-free
- SambalOelek, at will
- 1 lime
- Black pepper
- Coconut oil for frying

Directions

1. Dab the chicken breast with paper towels. Bring the pot with plenty of water and a little sea salt to the boil and cook the meat in it for about 20 minutes.
2. In the meantime, wash the zucchini, cut the ends, wash the carrots and peel thinly.
3. Use a vegetable peeler or a spiral cutter to cut long strips from the courgette and carrots.
4. Wash the chicory, remove the stalk and peel off the leaves.
5. Heat sesame oil in a pan, add the vegetable noodles and simmer over medium heat for about 5 minutes.
6. Add the chicory and cook for another 2-3 minutes. Halve and squeeze the lime.
7. Then season the vegetables with soy sauce, sambaloelek, approx. 1 tablespoon of lime juice, sea salt and black pepper.
8. Remove the cooked chicken breast fillets from the water, drain in a colander and pat dry a little.
9. Then cut into slices. Heat a pan with coconut oil. Put the meat in the pan and toss over a medium heat for about 4-5 minutes, deglaze with soy sauce.
10. Finally season with pepper and sea salt. Divide the vegetable noodles on two plates and serve with the meat.

Nutrition facts: Calories: 163 kcal Protein: 15.26 fat: 3.84 g Carbohydrates: 18.87 g

Grilled Steak Pinwheels

Prep time: 10 minutes

Cook time: 12 minutes

Serves: 4

Ingredients

- Beef flank steaks
- 2 Bacon strips
- 1/2 pound Fresh mushrooms
- 1 cup Green onions
- 1 cup Fresh basil
- 1/4 cup Minced chives, 2 tablespoons

Instructions

1. Flatten steaks to 1/4-inch thickness.
2. Mix bacon, mushrooms, onions, some basil, and the chives in a mixing bowl; spread over steaks.
3. Roll up the meat and protect it with the skewers.
4. Cut the rolls into 1/2- to 3/4-inch slices and secure with a toothpick.
5. Grill for about 4-6 minutes per side over medium-high heat till meat is cooked.
6. Take out the toothpicks.
7. Now serve it.

Nutritional Facts Fat: 12g, Net Carbs: 2g, Protein: 26g, Sodium: 250mg

Taco-stuffed Peppers

Prep time: 10 minutes

Cook time: 30 minutes

Serves: 4

Ingredients

- 1 pound 80/20 ground beef
- 1 tablespoon chili powder
- 2 teaspoons cumin
- 1 teaspoon garlic powder
- 1 teaspoon salt
- ¼ teaspoon ground black pepper
- 1 (10-ounce) can diced tomatoes and green chiles, drained
- 4 medium green bell peppers
- 1 cup shredded Monterey jack cheese, divided

Instructions

1. In a medium skillet over medium heat, brown the ground beef about 7–10 minutes. When no pink remains, drain the fat from the skillet.
2. Return the skillet to the stovetop and add chili powder, cumin, garlic powder, salt, and black pepper.
3. Add drained can of diced tomatoes and chiles to the skillet. Continue cooking 3–5 minutes. While the mixture is cooking, cut each bell pepper in half.
4. Remove the seeds and white membrane.
5. Spoon the cooked mixture evenly into each bell pepper and top with a ¼ cup cheese. Place stuffed peppers into the air fryer basket.
6. Adjust the temperature to 350°F and set the timer for 15 minutes.
7. When done, peppers will be fork tender and cheese will be browned and bubbling.
8. Serve warm.

Nutritional Facts: Calories: 346 Protein: 27.8 G Fiber: 3.5 G Net Carbohydrates: 7.2 G Fat: 19.1 G Sodium: 991 Mg Carbohydrates: 10.7 G Sugar: 4.9 G

Quinoa Cakes with Fresh Tomato–cilantro Sauce

Prep time: 1 hour

Cook time: 15/20 min

Serves: 4

Ingredients:

- 1½ cups Vegetable Stock or low-sodium vegetable broth
- 1 cup quinoa, rinsed
- ¼ teaspoon plus pinch of kosher salt, divided
- 4 ounces shredded reduced-fat Monterey Jack cheese (about 1 cup)
- 2 large egg whites
- ¼ cup plain dry breadcrumbs
- Pinch of ground cayenne
- 2¼ teaspoons canola oil, divided

- 1 large tomato, chopped
- 2 tablespoons chopped fresh cilantro
- 2 tablespoons thinly sliced scallions
- 2 teaspoons lime juice

Instructions:

1. Combine the stock, quinoa, and 1/4 teaspoon of the salt in a medium saucepan and bring to a boil over high heat.
2. Reduce the heat to low, cover, and simmer until the quinoa is tender, 12 to 15 minutes.
3. Transfer to a medium bowl to cool.
4. Add the Monterey Jack, egg whites, breadcrumbs, and cayenne to the quinoa and stir to mix well.
5. Brush a 1/4-cup measuring cup with 1/4 teaspoon of the oil.
6. Spoon the quinoa mixture into the cup, pressing until it is lightly packed.
7. Invert the quinoa cakes onto a large plate.
8. Cover and refrigerate 30 minutes.
9. Meanwhile, place the tomato, cilantro, scallions, lime juice, and the remaining pinch of salt in a food processor.
10. Pulse until coarsely chopped, but not pureed, 4 to 5 times.
11. Set the sauce aside.
12. Heat a large nonstick skillet over medium heat.
13. Add the remaining 2 teaspoons oil and tilt the pan to coat the bottom evenly.
14. Add the quinoa cakes and cook, turning once, until well browned, 3 to 4 minutes on each side.
15. Spoon the sauce evenly onto 4 plates, top evenly with the quinoa cakes, and serve at once.

Nutrition facts: 39 g carb, 317 cal, 12 g fat, 4 g sat fat, 20 mg chol, 3 g fib, 16 g pro, 475 mg sod

Shrimp Salad

Prep time: 15 minutes

Cook time: 35 minutes

Servings: 4

Ingredients:

- 1-pound shrimp, chopped and boiled and deveined
- 1 well boiled egg, chopped
- 1 tablespoon green pepper, chopped
- 1 tablespoon celery, chopped
- 2 tablespoons mayonnaise
- 1 tablespoon onion, chopped
- 1 teaspoon lemon juice
- ⅛ teaspoon tabasco or hot sauce
- ½ teaspoon chili powder
- ½ teaspoon dry mustard

Instructions:

1. Mix all ingredients except lettuce in a mixing bowl; mix well.
2. Refrigerate for 30 minutes.
3. Serving options include as a salad laid out on lettuce or as a sandwich.

Nutrition facts: 157 calories, 232 milligrams sodium, 0 grams trans-fat, 26 grams protein, 233 milligrams potassium, 234 milligrams cholesterol, 5 grams total fat

Summer Spinach Salad with Grilled Chicken and Creamy

Prep time: 30 min

Cook time: 15 min

Serves: 2

Ingredients Salad:

- 2 medium chicken breasts (about 1 lb)
- Kosher salt and black pepper
- 8 ounces fresh baby spinach
- 2 cups mixed, fresh berries (like blueberries, raspberries, blackberries and sliced strawberries)
- ¼ cup crumbled goat cheese
- ¼ cup toasted pecans

Creamy Berry Balsamic Dressing:

- ¼ cup olive oil
- ¼ cup balsamic vinegar
- 1 cup mixed, fresh berries (like blueberries, raspberries, blackberries and sliced strawberries)
- ¼ cup Stonyfield Organic Nonfat Greek yogurt
- 1-teaspoon Dijon mustard
- 2 teaspoons honey
- Salt and pepper

Instruction:

1. Heat a grill pan over medium high heat, brush with olive oil.
2. Season the chicken breasts with salt and pepper and add them to the skillet.
3. Cook 5-6 minutes per side.
4. Set aside.
5. For the dressing, blend all ingredients until smooth.
6. Season with salt and pepper to taste.
7. Place the spinach in a large bowl.
8. Cut the chicken into slices and arrange the slices on top.
9. Scatter the berries, goat cheese and pecans on top.
10. Serve the creamy berry balsamic dressing on the side.

Nutrition facts: values Energy 295 kcal / Protein 10.2 g / P (phosphorus) 106 mg / K (potassium) 197.5 mg / Na (sodium) 40.2 mg

Greek Style Quesadillas

Prep Time: 10 Minutes

Cook Time: 10 Minutes

Serves: 4

Ingredients:

- 4 Whole Wheat Tortillas
- 1 Cup Mozzarella Cheese, Shredded
- 1 Cup Fresh Spinach, Chopped
- 2 Tbsp Greek Yogurt
- 1 Egg, Beaten
- ¼ Cup Green Olives, Sliced
- 1 Tbsp Olive Oil
- 1/3 Cup Fresh Cilantro, Chopped

Instructions:

Creamy Penne

Prep Time: 10 Minutes

Cook Time: 25 Minutes

Serves: 4

Ingredients:

- ½ Cup Penne, Dried
- 9 Oz Chicken Fillet
- 1 Tsp Italian Seasoning
- 1 Tbsp Olive Oil
- 1 Tomato, Chopped
- 1 Cup Heavy Cream
- 1 Tbsp Fresh Basil, Chopped
- ½ Tsp Salt
- 2 Oz Parmesan, Grated
- 1 Cup Water, For Cooking

Instructions:

1. In The Bowl, Combine Together Mozzarella Cheese, Spinach, Yogurt, Egg, Olives, And Cilantro.
2. Then Pour Olive Oil in The Skillet.
3. Place One Tortilla in The Skillet and Spread It with Mozzarella Mixture.
4. Top It with The Second Tortilla And Spread It With Cheese Mixture Again.
5. Then Place the Third Tortilla and Spread It With All Remaining Cheese Mixture.
6. Cover It with The Last Tortilla and Fry It For 5 Minutes From Each Side Over The Medium Heat.

Nutrition facts: values Energy 295 kcal / Protein 10.2 g / P (phosphorus) 106 mg / K (potassium) 197.5 mg / Na (sodium) 40.2 mg

1. Pour Water In The Pan, Add Penne, And Boil It For 15 Minutes.
2. Then Drain Water.
3. Pour Olive Oil In The Skillet And Heat It Up.
4. Slice The Chicken Fillet And Put It In The Hot Oil.

5. Sprinkle Chicken with Italian Seasoning And Roast For 2 Minutes From Each Side.
6. Then Add Fresh Basil, Salt, Tomato, And Grated Cheese.
7. Stir Well.
8. Add Heavy Cream and Cooked Penne.
9. Cook The Meal for 5 Minutes More Over the Medium Heat.
10. Stir It from Time to Time.

Nutrition facts: Calories 388, Fat 23.4g, Fiber 0.2g, Carbs 17.6g, Protein 17.6g

Colourful Tuna Salad with Bocconcini

Prep Time: 5 Minutes

Cook Time: 40 Minutes

Serves: 3

Ingredients:

- 1 Green Bell Pepper, Sliced
- 2 Cans Tuna In Brine, Drained
- ¼ Tsp Black Peppercorns, Preferably Freshly Ground
- 1 Tbsp Oyster Sauce
- 1 Head Iceberg Lettuce
- 1 Tsp Pasilla Chili Pepper, Finely Chopped
- 2 Garlic Cloves, Minced
- 2 Tsps Peanut Butter
- ½ Cup Radishes, Sliced
- 1 Yellow Bell Pepper, Sliced
- ½ Cup Kalamata Olives, Pitted and Sliced
- ½ Cup Yellow Onion, Thinly Sliced
- 1 Tsp Olive Oil
- 8 Ounces Bocconcini
- 1 Cucumber, Sliced
- 1 Tomato, Diced
- 1 Tsp Champagne Vinegar

Instructions:

1. Mix Cucumbers, Iceberg Lettuce, Peppers, Onion, Tuna, Radishes, Tomatoes And Kalamata Olives In A Salad Container.
2. In A Small Mixing Dish, Thoroughly Mix Champagne Vinegar, Olive Oil, Peanut Butter, Oyster Sauce Black Peppercorns, And Garlic.
3. Include This Vinaigrette To The Salad Bowl; Ensure To Toss Until Everything Is Well Coated.
4. Now, Top with Bocconcini and Serve Well-Chilled. Bon Appétit!

Nutrition facts: Calories 273, Protein 34.2g, Fat 11.7g, Carbs 6.7g, Sugar 2.5g

Baked Eggplant Turkey

Prep Time: 10 Minutes

Cook Time: 50 Minutes

Serves: 6-8

Ingredients:

- ½ cup green pepper, chopped
- ½ cup onion, finely chopped
- 1 large eggplant
- 2 tbsps vegetable oil
- 2 cups plain breadcrumbs
- 1 large egg, slightly beaten
- 1-pound lean ground turkey
- ½ tsp red pepper, optional

Instructions:

1. Preheat An Oven To 350^0F.
2. Grease A Casserole Dish With Some Cooking Spray.
3. In Boiling Water, Cook Eggplant Until Fully Tender.
4. Drain And Mash Eggplant Well.
5. Take A Medium Saucepan Or Skillet, Add Oil. Heat Over Medium Heat.
6. Add Onion, Green Pepper, And Stir-Cook Until It Becomes Translucent And Softened.
7. Add Ground Meat And Stir-Cook Until Evenly Brown.
8. Mix In Eggplant, Egg, And Breadcrumbs. Season To Taste With Red Pepper.
9. Add The Mixture In A Casserole Dish And Bake For 35-45 Minutes

Until Meat Is Cooked To Satisfaction.
10. Serve Warm.

Nutrition facts: Calories 263, Fat 7g, Phosphorus 162mg, Potassium 373mg, Sodium 281mg, Carbohydrates 4g, Protein 14g

Turkey Sausages

Prep Time: 10 Minutes

Cook Time: 10 Minutes

Serves: 2

Ingredients:

- 1/4 teaspoon salt
- 1/8 teaspoon garlic powder
- 1/8 teaspoon onion powder
- One teaspoon fennel seed
- 1 pound 7% fat ground turkey

Instructions:

1. Press the fennel seed and put together turkey with fennel seed, garlic, onion powder, and salt in a small cup.
2. Cover the bowl and refrigerate overnight.
3. Prepare the turkey with seasoning into different portions with a circle form and press them into patties ready to be cooked.
4. Cook at medium heat until browned.
5. Cook it for 1 to 2 minutes per side and serve them hot.
6. Enjoy!

Nutrition facts: Calories: 55 Protein: 7 g Sodium: 70 mg Potassium: 105 mg Phosphorus: 75 mg

Baked Garlic Lemon Salmon

Prep Time: 5 minutes

Cook time: 15 minutes

Serves: 4

Ingredients:
- 3 tablespoons lemon juice
- 4 medium-sized salmon fillets
- ¼ cup unsalted butter, melted
- 2 cloves garlic, minced
- A handful of parsley, finely chopped
- Salt and pepper to taste

Instructions
1. Preheat the oven to 400°F (200°C).
2. Line a baking dish or tray with tin foil; grease with some cooking spray.
3. Place the salmon fillets over the baking dish.
4. Add the butter, garlic, lemon juice, salt and pepper to a mixing bowl.
5. Mix well.
6. Brush the salmon fillets with the butter sauce, reserving some sauce.
7. Bake for around 15 minutes, or until the salmon is easy to flake.
8. Bake for 2–3 minutes more if needed.
9. Brush with the reserved sauce and sprinkle some lemon juice on top.
10. Serve with chopped parsley on top.

Nutrition facts: Calories 350 Fat 25 g Total carbs 2 g Sugar 0.5 g, Protein 28.5 g Sodium 68 mg

Hearty Pumpkin Chicken Soup

Prep Time: 15 minutes
Cook Time: 35 minutes
Servings 6

Ingredients

- 1 small onion, thinly sliced
- 2 cloves garlic, minced
- 1 pound chicken breast, thinly sliced
- 1 tablespoon vegetable oil or coconut oil
- 1 medium zucchini, diced
- 1-inch piece ginger, peeled and minced
- ¾ pound pumpkin, cubed into ½-inch pieces
- 1 small chili or jalapeno pepper, seeded and thinly sliced
- 1 red bell pepper, seeded and thinly sliced
- 2 cups chicken broth
- 1 (14-ounce) can light coconut milk A handful of cilantro leaves Juice of 1 lime
- Salt and pepper to taste

Directions

1. Season the chicken slices with salt and pepper.
2. Heat the oil over medium-high heat in a large cooking pot.
3. Add the chicken and stir cook for 4–5 minutes to evenly brown.
4. Add the onion, ginger, and garlic and stir cook for 2–3 minutes until softened and translucent.
5. Add the zucchini and cubed pumpkin; stir well.
6. Add the chicken broth, coconut milk, bell pepper, chili or jalapeno pepper, and lime juice; stir again.
7. Bring to a boil, cover, and simmer over low heat for about 20 minutes, until the pumpkin is cooked well and softened.
8. Season with additional salt and pepper, if required.
9. Serve warm with cilantro leaves on top.

10. Note: You can store leftovers in an airtight container in the refrigerator for up to 3–4 days.
11. Simply re-heat in a cooking pot and serve.

Nutrition facts: Calories 231 Fat 13 g Total carbs 11.5 g Sugar 5 g, Protein 17 g Sodium 1207 mg

Colorful sweet potato salad

Prep Time: 5 minutes
Cook Time: 30 minutes
Servings: 4
Ingredients

- 450 g sweet potato
- Sea salt and black pepper, curry powder, to taste
- 1 ½ tbsp. olive oil
- 100 g baby spinach
- ½ organic lemon
- 30 g of walnuts
- ½ organic apple, green
- ½ teaspoon maple syrup
- 1 tbsp. vegetable stock
- 2 tbsp. quinoa, puffed, approx. 15 g
- ½ handful of chive flowers

Directions

1. Preheat the oven to 200 degrees (convection). Line a baking sheet with parchment paper.
2. Peel the sweet potato and cut into bite-sized pieces.
3. Mix with sea salt, black pepper, curry and 1 tbsp. oil and place on the baking tray, cook for about 20 minutes, turning occasionally, then leave to cool.
4. In the meantime, clean, wash and spin-dry the spinach. Halve the lemon, squeeze out the juice. Chop walnuts.
5. Wash the apple, cut into quarters and remove the core, cut into bite-sized pieces and drizzle with a little lemon juice.
6. For the dressing, stir together lemon juice, maple syrup, sea salt, pepper and oil vigorously.

7. Finally, put all the ingredients in a bowl and mix with the dressing. Then divide the salad on two plates, sprinkle the quinoa on top and garnish with the chives flowers.
8. Note: Quinoa (puffed) is already available in many supermarkets, but also in health food stores and health food stores.

Nutrition facts: Calories: 211 kcal Protein: 5.49 g Fat: 14.41 g Carbohydrates: 19.38 g

Barbecue Pork Loin

Prep Time: 10 minutes, plus 20 minutes marinating time
Cook Time: 35 minutes
Servings: 6
Ingredients
- 1½ pounds boneless pork sirloin roast
- 1 cup white vinegar
- 3 small garlic cloves, pressed
- 1 tbsp. creole seasoning
- ½ tsp smoked paprika
- ½ tsp cayenne pepper
- ½ cup chicken broth (here) or store-bought low-sodium chicken broth, plus more as needed
- ½ cup Barbecue Sauce, plus more for serving

Directions
1. Preheat the oven to 400°F.
2. In a medium bowl, combine the pork, vinegar, and garlic.
3. Set aside to marinate for 10 minutes.
4. Remove the pork from the marinade, shaking off any remaining vinegar, and transfer to a rimmed baking sheet.
5. Massage the pork all over with the Creole seasoning, paprika, and cayenne.
6. Cover and set aside for 20 minutes. In a Dutch oven, bring the broth to a simmer over high heat.
7. Add the pork and cook for 2 to 3 minutes per side, or until lightly browned. If the broth runs low, to keep the pork moist, add ¼ cup when turning.

8. Cover the pot, transfer to the oven, and cook for 30 minutes or until the pork is opaque.
9. Cover with the barbecue sauce, return to the oven, and cook for 5 to 7 minutes, or until a nice crust forms on the exterior.
10. Transfer the pork to a cutting board. Let rest for 5 to 10 minutes.
11. Slice the pork and serve with extra barbecue sauce.

Nutrition facts: Calories: 204 Total fat: 7 g Cholesterol: 75 mg Sodium: 134 mg

Ginger Halibut Bites

Prep time: 15 minutes
Cook time: 15 minutes
Serves: 4
Ingredients
- Lemon juice
- 4 teaspoons Halibut fillets
- 4 Minced gingerroot
- 1 teaspoon Salt
- 3/4 teaspoon Pepper
- 1/4 teaspoon Water
- 1/2 cup Brussels sprouts
- 10 ounces Red pepper flakes
- 1 tablespoon Canola oil
- 1 tablespoon Garlic cloves
- 5 Sesame oil
- 2 tablespoons Soy sauce
- 2 tablespoons

Instructions
1. Brush the halibut fillets with lemon juice.
2. Toss with some minced ginger, 1/4 teaspoon of salt, and freshly ground pepper.
3. Place the fish down from the skin side onto an oiled grill shelf.
4. Grill, covered, over medium heat for 6-8 mins, till the fish starts to flake effortlessly with a fork. Boil the water in a skillet over medium-high heat.
5. Stir in the Brussels sprouts with pepper flakes and any remaining salt if necessary.
6. Cook, covered, for 5-7 minutes, or until the vegetables are soft.
7. Meanwhile, heat oil into a skillet over a medium flame.

8. Cook until the garlic is golden brown. Using paper towels, drain it.
9. Drizzle halibut with sesame oil and some soy sauce.
10. Now serve with Brussels sprouts and fried garlic.
11. Serve with some lemon slices if needed.

Nutritional Facts Fat: 12g, Net Carbs: 7g, Protein: 24g, Sodium: 701mg

Sirloin Steak With Tomato & Pepper

Prep time: 15 minutes
Cook time: 35 minutes
Serves: 6

Ingredients
- Whole wheat flour 1/2 cup
- Salt,
- 3/4 teaspoon Pepper,
- Sirloin steak, chopped, 1-1/2 pounds
- Canola oil 3-4 tablespoons
- Chopped onion 1
- Chopped garlic clove
- 1 Chopped tomatoes,
- 30 ounces Chopped green pepper,
- 2 Beef broth,
- 3-4 tablespoons Worcestershire sauce,
- 1.5 teaspoons Cooked rice, 1 bowl

Instructions
1. Combine the first 3 ingredients inside a large mixing bowl.
2. Add them with the beef, one at a time.
3. Mix gently to coat the beef with the mixture.
4. Warm the oil inside a Dutch oven at medium-high temperature.
5. Cook the beef in batches.
6. Include onion; bake and stir for 4-5 minutes, or until the onion is tender.
7. Now in a skillet, include garlic; cook for 1 minute.
8. Add tomatoes and again cook for few minutes.
9. Reduce the flame.
10. Now transfer the meat to skillet and Simmer, covered, for 11-16 minutes, or until the meat is tender.

11. Whisk in green peppers, beef broth, and sauce; cook covered for 11-15 minutes until the peppers are soft. Serve with rice.

Nutritional Facts Fat: 12g, Net Carbs: 17g, Protein: 27g, Sodium: 552mg

Italian Chicken

Prep time: 10 minutes
Cook time: 30 minutes
Serves: 4
Ingredients
- 5 chicken thighs
- 1 tbsp. olive oil
- 1/4 cup parmesan; grated
- 1/2 cup sun dried tomatoes
- 2 garlic cloves; minced
- 1 tbsp. thyme; chopped.
- 1/2 cup heavy cream
- 3/4 cup chicken stock
- 1 tsp. red pepper flakes; crushed
- 2 tbsp. basil; chopped
- Salt and black pepper to the taste

Instructions

1. Season chicken with salt and pepper, rub with half of the oil, place in your preheated air fryer at 350 °F and cook for 4 minutes.
2. Meanwhile; heat up a pan with the rest of the oil over medium high heat, add thyme garlic, pepper flakes, sun dried tomatoes, heavy cream, stock, parmesan, salt and pepper; stir, bring to a simmer, take off heat and transfer to a dish that fits your air fryer.
3. Add chicken thighs on top, introduce in your air fryer and cook at 320 °F, for 12 minutes.
4. Divide among plates and serve with basil sprinkled on top.

Nutritional Facts: Calories: 272; Fat: 9; Fiber: 12; Carbs: 37; Protein: 23

Parmesan-Topped Acorn Squash

Prep Time: 8 minutes
Cook Time: 20 minutes
Serves: 4

Ingredients

- 1 acorn squash (about 1 pound)
- 1 tablespoon extra-virgin olive oil
- 1 teaspoon dried sage leaves, crumbled
- ¼ teaspoon freshly grated nutmeg
- 1/8 teaspoon kosher salt
- 1/8 teaspoon freshly ground black pepper
- 2 tablespoons freshly grated Parmesan cheese

Instructions

1. Chop acorn squash in half lengthwise and remove the seeds. Cut each half in half for a total of 4 wedges. Snap off the stem if it's easy to do.
2. In a small bowl, combine the olive oil, sage, nutmeg, salt, and pepper. Brush the cut sides of the squash with the olive oil mixture.
3. Fill 1 cup of water into the electric pressure cooker and insert a wire rack or trivet.
4. Place the squash on the trivet in a single layer, skin-side down.
5. Set the lid of the pressure cooker on sealing.
6. Cook on high pressure for 20 minutes.
7. Once done, press Cancel and quick release the pressure.
8. Once the pin drops, open it.
9. Carefully remove the squash from the pot, sprinkle with the Parmesan, and serve.

Nutritional Facts: 85 Calories 12g Carbohydrates 2g Fiber

Fish & Chip Traybake

Prep time: 30/40 min
Cook time: 35 min
Serving: 4
Ingredients:
- 2 large sweet potatoes, cut into thin wedges
- 1 tbsp rapeseed oil
- 4 tbsp fat-free natural yogurt
- 2 tbsp low-fat mayonnaise
- 3 cornichons, finely chopped,
- 1 tbsp of the brine
- 1 shallot, finely chopped
- 1 tbsp finely chopped dill, plus extra to serve
- 300g frozen peas
- 50ml milk
- 1 tbsp finely chopped mint
- 4 cod or Pollock loin fillets
- 1 lemon, cut into wedges, to serve

Instructions:
1. Heat the oven to 220C/200C fan/gas Toss the sweet potatoes with the oil and a little seasoning on a baking sheet and roast for 20 minutes.
2. Combine the yoghurt, mayonnaise, cornichons and reserved brine, shallots and dill with 1 tbsp cold water on the side.
3. Place the peas in a saucepan with the milk, bring to the boil and cook for 5 minutes.
4. Blend the mixture until coarsely pureed.
5. Stir in the mint and season to taste.
6. Set aside.
7. Add the cod or pollock to the pan with the sweet potatoes, season and bake for 10-15 minutes more or until cooked through.
8. Heat the pea mixture.
9. Sprinkle on some dill and serve the baking dish with the yogurt tartare and mushy peas.

Nutrition facts: 206 calories, 184 milligrams sodium, 6 grams trans-fat, 20 grams protein, 4g fat

Pork in Chinese

Prep time: 10 min

Cook time: 7/8 min

Serves 2

Ingredients:

- pork lean meat 50 g
- frozen vegetables Chinese mixture 100 g
- quality vegetable oil 15 g
- solamyl 5 g (potato powder)

Instruction

1. We clean the meat, cut it into strips, wrap it in solamyl.
2. Fry the meat in a hot pan.
3. Then add vegetables, a small amount of water and stew.
4. Lightly salt.

Nutrition facts: values Energy 295 kcal / Protein 10.2 g / P (phosphorus) 106 mg / K (potassium) 197.5 mg / Na (sodium) 40.2 mg

Coconut Chicken Curry

Prep Time: 10 Minutes

Cook Time: 40 Minutes

Serves: 6

Ingredients:

- 1 Small Sweet Onion
- 2 Tsps Minced Garlic
- 1 Tsp Grated Ginger
- 3 Tbsps Olive Oil
- 6 Boneless, Skinless Chicken Thighs
- 1 Tbsp Curry Powder
- ¾ Cup of Water
- ¼ Cup of Coconut Milk
- 2 Tbsps Cilantro, Chopped

Instructions:

1. Place A Medium Saucepan or Skillet On Medium Heat, Add 2 Tablespoons Oil.
2. Add Chicken and Stir-Cook Until Evenly Brown, About 8-10 Minutes.
3. Set Aside.

4. Add Remaining Oil.
5. Add Onion, Ginger, Garlic, And Stir-Cook Until Softened, About 3-4 Minutes.
6. Mix In Curry Powder, Water And Coconut Milk.
7. Add Chicken, Stir The Mixture And Boil It.
8. Cover And Simmer The Mixture Over Low Heat For Another 25 Minutes Until Chicken Is Tender.
9. Serve Warm With Cilantro On Top.

Nutrition facts: Calories 258, Fat 13g, Phosphorus 151mg, Potassium 242mg, Sodium 86mg, Carbohydrates 2g, Protein 25g

Chicken and Veggie Soup

Prep Time: 15 Minutes

Cook Time: 25 Minutes

Serves: 8

Ingredients:

- 4 - cups cooked and chopped chicken
- 7 - cups reduced-sodium chicken broth
- 1 - pound froze white corn
- 1 - medium onion diced
- 4 - cloves garlic minced
- 2 - carrots peeled and diced
- 2 - celery stalks chopped
- 2 - teaspoons oregano
- 2 - teaspoon curry powder
- ½ - teaspoon black pepper

Instructions:

1. Include all fixings into the moderate cooker.
2. Cook on LOW for 8hours Serve over cooked white rice.

Nutrition facts: Calories: 220 Fat: 7g Protein: 24g Carbs: 19g

Seafood and Andouille Medley

Prep Time: 5 Minutes

Cook Time: 40 Minutes

Serves: 3

Ingredients:

- 2 Andouille Sausages,
- Cut Crosswise Into ½-Inch-Thick Slices
- ½ Stick Butter, Melted
- 2 Tomatoes, Pureed
- 2 Tbsps Fresh Cilantro, Chopped
- ½ Pound Skinned Sole, Cut into Chunks
- 1/3 Cup Dry White Wine
- 1 Shallot, Chopped
- 2 Garlic Cloves, Finely Minced
- 1 Tbsp Oyster Sauce
- 3/4 Cup Clam Juice
- 20 Sea Scallops

Instructions:

1. Dissolve the butter in a heavy-bottomed pot over medium-high heat.
2. Heat the sausages until no longer pink; set aside.
3. Sauté the garlic and shallots in the same pan until they are softened; set aside.
4. Include the oyster sauce, pureed tomatoes, clam juice and wine; simmer for another 12 minutes.
5. Add the scallops, skinned sole and sausages.
6. Let it simmer, partially covered, for another 6 minutes.
7. Enjoy garnished with fresh cilantro. Bon appétit!

Nutrition facts: Calories 481, Protein 46.6g, Fat 26.9g, Carbs 5g, Sugar 1.1g

Chicken and Veggie Soup

Prep Time: 15 Minutes

Cook Time: 25 Minutes

Serves: 8

Ingredients:

- 4 - cups cooked and chopped chicken
- 7 - cups reduced-sodium chicken broth
- 1 - pound froze white corn
- 1 - medium onion diced
- 4 - cloves garlic minced
- 2 - carrots peeled and diced
- 2 - celery stalks chopped
- 2 - teaspoons oregano
- 2 - teaspoon curry powder
- ½ - teaspoon black pepper

Instructions:

3. Include all fixings into the moderate cooker.
4. Cook on LOW for 8hours Serve over cooked white rice.

Nutrition facts: Calories: 220 Fat:7g Protein: 24g Carbs: 19g

Ground Lamb with Peas

Prep Time: 15 Minutes

Cook Time: 55 Minutes

Serves: 4

Ingredients:

- One tablespoon coconut oil
- Three dried red chilies
- 1 (2-inch) cinnamon stick
- Three green cardamom pods
- ½ teaspoon cumin seeds
- One medium red onion, chopped
- 1 (¾-inch) piece fresh ginger, minced
- Four garlic cloves, minced
- 1½ teaspoons ground coriander
- ½ teaspoon garam masala
- ½ teaspoon ground cumin
- ½ teaspoon ground turmeric
- ¼ teaspoon ground nutmeg

- Two bay leaves
- 1-pound lean ground lamb
- ½ cup Roma tomatoes, chopped
- 1-1½ cups water
- 1 cup fresh green peas, shelled
- Two tablespoons plain Greek yogurt, whipped
- ¼ cup fresh cilantro, sliced
- Salt and freshly ground black pepper

Instructions:

1. In a Dutch oven, melt coconut oil on medium-high heat.
2. Add red chilies, cinnamon sticks, cardamom pods, and cumin seeds and sauté for around thirty seconds.
3. Add onion and sauté for about 3-4 minutes.
4. Add ginger, garlic cloves, and spices and sauté for around thirty seconds.
5. Add lamb and cook approximately 5 minutes.
6. Add tomatoes and cook approximately 10 min.
7. Stir in water and green peas and cook, covered approximately 25-thirty minutes.
8. Stir in yogurt, cilantro, salt, and black pepper and cook for around 4-5 minutes. Serve hot.

Nutrition facts: Calories: 430 Fat: 10g Carbohydrates: 22g Fiber: 6g Protein: 26g

Asian-Style Pan-Fried Chicken

Prep Time: 20 Minutes

Cook Time: 25 Minutes

Serves: 4

Ingredients:

- 12 ounces boneless, skinless chicken thighs, fat removed, cut into 2 or 3 pieces each
- One teaspoon low-sodium soy sauce
- One teaspoon dry rice wine
- 1-inch piece ginger, minced
- ½ cup cornstarch
- Three teaspoons canola oil, divided

- One lemon, cut into wedges

Instructions:

1. In a medium bowl, combine the chicken, soy sauce, rice wine, and ginger.
2. Toss and let sit for 15 minutes.
3. Toss the chicken again, and drain the liquid from the bowl.
4. One at a time, put the chicken pieces in the cornstarch to coat.
5. In a medium skillet over medium-high heat, heat 1½ teaspoons of oil, add half of the chicken to the pan, and cook until golden brown on one side, about 3 to 5 minutes.
6. Flip and continue to cook on the opposite side until the chicken is cooked through and is golden brown.
7. Transfer the chicken to a plate wrinkled with paper towels to cool.
8. Add the remaining 1½ teaspoons of oil, and repeat the cooking process with the remaining chicken thighs.
9. Serve garnished with lemon wedges.

Nutrition facts: Calories: 198 Total Fat: 7g Cholesterol: 71mg Carbohydrates: 16g Fiber: 0g Protein: 17g Phosphorus: 148mg Potassium: 218mg Sodium: 119mg

Dessert

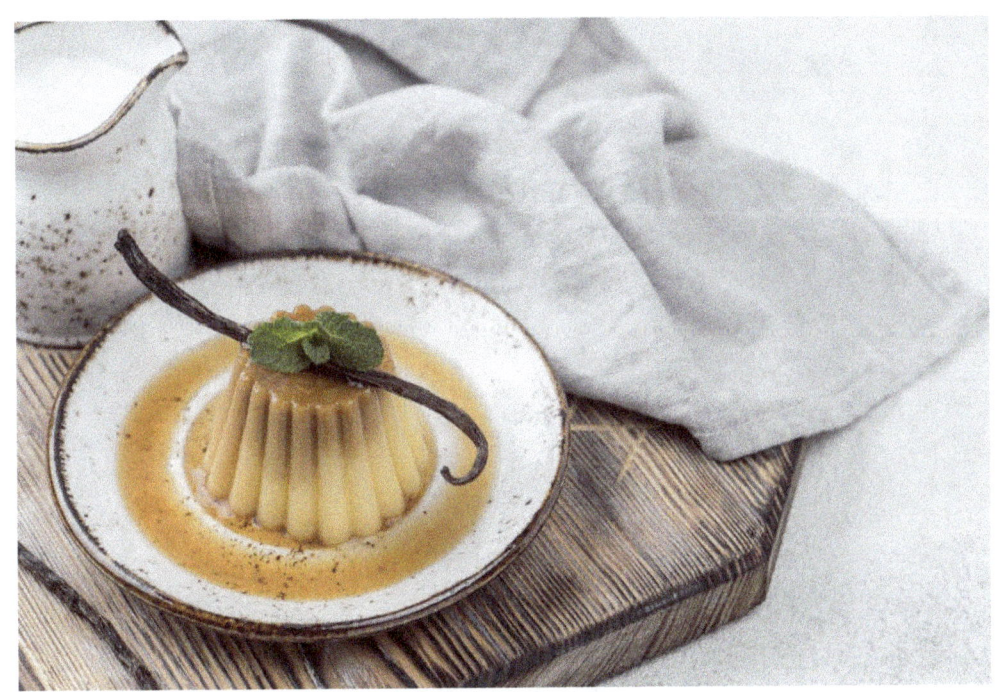

Strawberry Lemon Muffins

Preparation Time: 8 Minutes
Cooking Time: 30 Minutes
Servings: 6
Ingredients:

- 6 eggs
- 2 ¼ cups almond flour
- 1 cup strawberry, chopped
- ¼ cup coconut flour
- ¼ cup sweetener
- ¼ cup sugar-free artificial honey
- 1 teaspoon vanilla
- ½ teaspoon salt
- 2 tablespoons butter
- 1 teaspoon baking soda

Streusel Ingredients:

- ¼ cup almond flour
- 1/3 cup chopped pecans (or any other nuts)
- 1 tablespoon sugar-free honey
- 2 tablespoons sweetener
- 2 tablespoons butter, softened
- ½ teaspoon cinnamon

Instructions:

1. Preheat the oven to 350°F.
2. Line a 12-cup muffin tin with paper liners.
3. In a large mixing bowl, combine almond flour, coconut flour, sweetener, baking soda, and salt.
4. Slowly add in eggs, honey, butter, and vanilla.
5. Make sure all ingredients are blended thoroughly.
6. Fold in strawberries, making sure not to puree them.
7. In a separate bowl, mix streusel ingredients and set aside.
8. Pour the batter evenly among the muffin liners.
9. Lightly sprinkle with streusel topping.
10. Bake for 25-30 minutes.

Nutrition facts: Calories: 127 Total Carbs: 14g Fat: 3g Protein: 19g 77. Low Carb

English Muffins

Preparation Time: 11 Minutes
Cooking Time: 28 Minutes
Servings: 6
Ingredients:
- 1 egg
- 1 tablespoon coconut flour
- 1 teaspoon psyllium husk powder
- 1 tablespoon water
- Pinch of baking powder
- Pinch of salt

Instructions:
1. Whisk together the egg, olive oil, and water in a mug or a small microwavable bowl or ramekin
2. Add the coconut flour, psyllium husk, baking powder, and salt, and whisk until there are no lumps
3. Microwave on high for about 1 ½-2 minutes until it is cooked through. Serve and enjoy!

Nutrition facts: Calories: 124 Total Carbs: 12g Fat: 8g Protein: 19g Chapter 6.

Chocolate Cookies

Preparation Time: 11 Minutes
Cooking Time: 25 Minutes
Servings: 6
Ingredients:
- 1 cup all-purpose flour
- 1/4 teaspoon baking soda
- 1/4 cup light margarine
- 1/2 cup granulated Splenda
- 1/3 cup unsweetened cocoa powder
- 1/4 cup packed Splenda brown sugar blend
- 1/4 cup buttermilk
- 1 teaspoon vanilla extract
- 1 tablespoon confectioner's sugar

Instructions:
1. In a small bowl, combine flour and baking soda; set aside.
2. In a medium saucepan, melt margarine; remove from the heat.
3. Stir in granulated Splenda, cocoa powder, and Splenda brown sugar blend.
4. Stir in buttermilk and vanilla.
5. Stir in flour mixture just until combined.

6. Cover and chill dough for 1 hour; the dough should be stiff.

7. Preheat the oven to 350°F.

8. Lightly coat two baking sheets with cooking spray.

9. Drop the dough by rounded teaspoons onto baking sheets.

10. Bake 8 to 10 minutes, or until edges are set.

11. Cool 1 minute, then transfer to a wire rack to cool completely.

12. Sprinkle with confectioner's sugar.

Nutrition facts: Calories: 66 Fat: 2g Carbohydrates: 12g Protein: 1g

Coconut Keto Bombs

Preparation time: 15 minutes
Cooking time: 0 minutes
Servings 14
Ingredients:

- 1 and ½ cups of walnuts or any type of nuts of your choice
- ½ Cup of shredded coconut
- ¼ Cup of coconut butter + 1 additional tablespoon of extra coconut butter
- 2 Tablespoons of almond butter
- 2 Tablespoons of chia seeds
- 2 Tablespoons of flax meal
- 2 Tablespoons of hemp seeds
- 1 Teaspoon of cinnamon
- ½ Teaspoon of vanilla bean powder
- ¼ Teaspoon of kosher salt
- 2 Tablespoons of cacao nibs

For the chocolate drizzle

- 1 Oz of unsweetened chocolate, chopped
- ½ Teaspoon of coconut oil

Instructions:

1. In the mixing bowl of your food processor, combine the walnuts with the coconut butter; the almond butter, the chia seeds, the flax meal, the hemp seeds, the cinnamon, the vanilla bean powder, the shredded coconut and the chopped; then drizzle with the coconut oil.
2. Pulse your ingredients for about 1 to 2 minutes or until the mixture starts breaking down.
3. Keep processing your mixture until it starts to stick together; but just be careful not to over mix.
4. Add in the cacao nibs and pulse until your ingredients.
5. With a small cookie scoop or simply with a tablespoon, divide the mixture into pieces of equal size.
6. Use both your hands to toll the mixture into balls; then arrange it over a platter. Store the balls in an airtight container or place it in the freezer for about 15 minutes.
7. Serve and enjoy your delicious balls!

Nutrition facts: Calories: 164| Fat: 14 g | Carbohydrates: 5.9g | Fiber: 2g |Protein: 4 g

Pecan Coffee Cake

Prep time: 20 min
Cook time: 40 min
Serves 4
Ingredients:

- 1/2 cup margarine, softened
- 1/2 cup Splenda
- 3 eggs
- 1/2 cup almond milk
- 1 teaspoon vanilla extract
- 1/2 cup sugar-free caramel sauce, divided
- 1/2 cup chopped pecans, divided
- 3 cups almond flour
- 1 teaspoon baking powder
- 1 teaspoon baking soda
- 1/2 teaspoon salt

Instructions:

1. Preheat oven to 325F, coat a Bundt pan with cooking spray.

2. In a medium bowl, combine almond flour, baking powder, baking soda, and salt; mix well and set aside.
3. In a large bowl, beat margarine and Splenda until frothy.
4. Beat in eggs, milk, and vanilla.
5. Add flour mixture and beat until well mixed.
6. Pour half the batter in bundt pan, drizzle with half the caramel sauce, and sprinkle with half the pecans.
7. Swirl with a knife.
8. Pour remaining batter over nuts.
9. Bake 35-40 minutes, or until toothpick comes out clean.
10. Let cool 15 to 20 minutes then drizzle with remaining caramel sauce and sprinkle with remaining pecans.

Nutrition facts: 232 calories; 20g fat; 7g carbohydrates; 6g protein; per 1/16 of recipe

Jalapeno and Cheddar Muffins

Prep Time: 9 Minutes
Cook Time: 35 Minutes
Servings: 8
Ingredients:
- cups finely diced raw cauliflower
- 2 tablespoons minced jalapeno
- 2 eggs, beaten
- 2 tablespoons melted butter
- 1/3 cup grated parmesan cheese
- 1 cup grated mozzarella cheese
- 1 cup grated cheddar cheese
- 1 tablespoon dried onion flakes
- ¼ teaspoon salt
- ¼ teaspoon black pepper
- ½ teaspoon garlic powder
- ½ teaspoon baking powder
- ¼ cup coconut flour

Instructions:
1. Preheat the oven to 375°F.
2. Combine the cauliflower, jalapeno, eggs, add melted butter in a medium bowl.
3. Add the grated cheeses and mix well.

4. Stir in the onion flakes, salt, pepper, garlic powder, baking powder, and coconut flour until thoroughly combined.
5. Divide the batter evenly between 12 greased muffin cups.
6. Bake for 30 minutes or until golden brown.
7. Turn off the oven and leave the muffins inside for about an hour.
8. Remove from the oven.
9. Cool on a wire rack.
10. Serve and enjoy!

Nutrition facts: Calories: 130 Total Carbs: 13g Fat: 6g Protein: 19g 74. Low Carb

Honey Raisin Cookies

Prep Time: 11 Minutes

Cook Time: 29 Minutes

Servings: 6

Ingredients:
- 1/2 cup butter, softened
- 1/2 cup honey
- 1 egg
- 1 teaspoon vanilla
- 1 cup whole wheat flour
- 1 teaspoon baking powder
- 1/4 teaspoon salt
- 1/2 cup oats
- 1/2 cup raisins
- 1/2 cup chopped walnuts

Instructions:
1. Combine the first four ingredients and mix well.
2. Combine the next four ingredients and add to the honey-butter mixture.
3. Add the raisins and chopped walnuts.
4. Bake at 350°F for 12-15 minutes or until just lightly golden brown.

Nutrition facts: Calories: 227 Fat: 12g Carbohydrates: 28g Protein: 4g

Sweet Potato Bread

Preparation time: 15 minutes
Cooking time: 45 minutes
Servings 4
Ingredients:
- 1 large peeled and diced sweet potato
- 1 Tbsp of ground flaxseeds
- 3 Tbsp of water
- 2 and ½ cups of almond flour
- 1 Teaspoon of dried thyme
- 1 Teaspoon of fresh chopped rosemary
- ½ Teaspoon of sea salt
- 2 Tbsp of extra-virgin olive oil

Instructions:
1. Preheat your oven to around 350 F.
2. Steam your sweet potatoes into a steamer basket in an instant pot or boil steam it in a steamer basket above the stove on top of boiling water for around 6 to 9 minutes.
3. Mix the flax seeds with water in a deep bowl and set it aside for around 10 minutes.
4. Mix again very well and mash the cooked potatoes with a potato masher or with a fork.
5. Add the rest of the ingredients and then add the rest of the ingredients and mix all the ingredients together very well.
6. Form the dough from your mixture and transfer your dough to a lined parchment and roll the dough with a rolling pin into around ½ inch of thickness.
7. Bake the dough for about 40 to 45 minutes.
8. Once the bread becomes brown, remove it from the oven and set it aside to cool down for around 20 minutes.
9. Cut the bread into rectangles.
10. Serve and enjoy!

Nutrition facts: Calories: 100 | Fat: 3 g | Carbohydrates: 11g | Fiber: 1 g |Protein: 4.9 g

Raspberry and Cashew Balls

Preparation time: 15 minutes
Cooking time: 0 minutes
Servings 14
Ingredients:
- 1⅓ Cup of raw cashews or almonds
- ¼ Cup of cashew or almond butter
- 2 Tablespoons of coconut oil
- 2 Pitted Medjool dates, pre-soaked into hot water for about 10 minutes
- ½ Teaspoon of vanilla extract
- ¼ Teaspoon of kosher salt
- ½ Cup of freeze-dried and lightly crashed raspberries
- 1 Cup of chopped dark chocolate

Instructions:
1. In a high-powered blender or a Vitamix; combine the cashews or almonds with the butter, the coconut oil, the Medjool dates, the vanilla extract and the salt and pulse on a high speed for about 1 to 2 minutes or until the batter starts sticking together.
2. Pulse in the dried raspberries and the dark chocolate until your get a thick mixture.
3. With a tablespoon or a small cookie scoop, divide the mixture into balls of equal size.
4. Arrange the balls in a container or a zip-top bag in a refrigerator for about 2 weeks or just serve and enjoy your delicious cashew balls!

Nutrition facts; Calories: 108.2| Fat: 7.4 g | Carbohydrates: 5.9g | Fiber: 1.3g |Protein: 3 g

Conclusion

Diabetes mellitus is growing in epidemic proportions, leading to devastating complications if not treated well. There are many challenges in the successful treatment of diabetes mellitus because of the personal and economic costs incurred in diabetes care.

Diabetes is a disease in which blood glucose, or blood sugar, levels are too high. Glucose comes from the foods you eat. Insulin is a hormone that helps glucose enter cells to give them energy. With type 1 diabetes, your body doesn't make insulin. Diabetes, the major component of chronic metabolic diseases, not only lowers your quality of life and greatly increases your medical bills, but it also significantly increases disease-related deaths. Diabetes has become one of the leading diseases leading to death.

If not controlled, diabetes can damage the heart, blood vessels, eyes, kidneys and nerves. That's why it's so important to get screened for diabetes and take steps to prevent it if you are identified as being at increased risk. Diabetes is a disease that occurs when your blood sugar, or glucose, is too high.

Control your diabetes control your life....

The healthy way to eat the foods you love

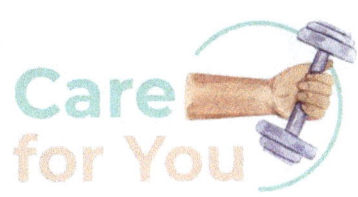
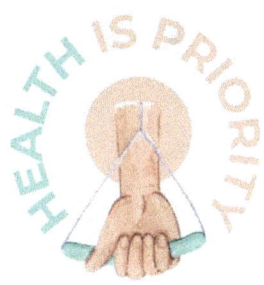
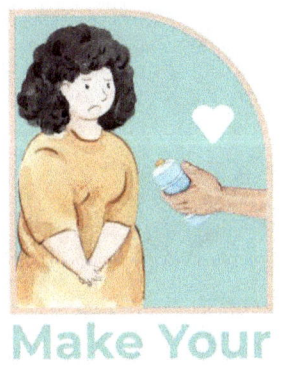
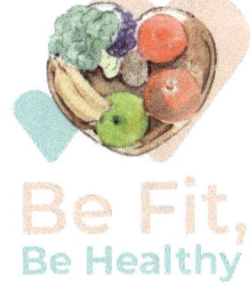

www.ingramcontent.com/pod-product-compliance
Lightning Source LLC
Chambersburg PA
CBHW081417080526
44589CB00016B/2563